Guiding Clients in Recovery From Psychological Trauma

Copyright © 2017 by J. Douglas Bremner

ISBN 978-0-9908650-8-7

Printed in the United States of America

While the authors have made every effort to provide accurate telephone numbers and Internet addresses at the time of publication, neither the publisher nor the authors assume any responsibility for errors or for changes that occur after publication. As well, the publisher does not have any control over and does not assume responsibility for authors' or third-party websites or their content.

I0102854

ALSO by DR. J. DOUGLAS BREMNER

TRAUMA, MEMORY AND DISSOCIATION (Progress in Psychiatry, Edited with C. Marmar) American Psychiatric Press, 1998.

POSTTRAUMATIC STRESS DISORDER: A Comprehensive Text (Edited with P. Saigh). Allyn & Bacon, 1999.

BRAIN IMAGING HANDBOOK, W.W. Norton & Company, 2005.

DOES STRESS DAMAGE THE BRAIN? UNDERSTANDING TRAUMA-RELATED DISORDERS FROM A MIND-BODY PERSPECTIVE. W.W. Norton & Company, 2002.

BEFORE YOU TAKE THAT PILL: *Why the Drug Industry May Be Bad for Your Health: Risks and Side Effects You Won't Find on the Label of Commonly Prescribed Drugs, Vitamins, and Supplements*, Penguin Press / Avery Trade, 2008.

THE GOOSE THAT LAID THE GOLDEN EGG: Accutane, the Truth that Had to be Told. Right Publishing, 2011., 2nd Edition from Laughing Cow Books, 2014.

THE FASTEST GROWING RELIGION ON EARTH: How Genealogy Captured the Brains and Imaginations of Americans. Laughing Cow Books, 2013.

A FRESH LOOK AT GREED. Laughing Cow Books, 2013.

YOU CAN'T JUST SNAP OUT OF IT: *The True Path to Recovery From Psychological Trauma*, Laughing Cow Books, 2014.

More information about Dr. Bremner's books is at <u>dougbremner.com</u>

Table of Contents

GUIDING CLIENTS IN RECOVERY FROM PSYCHOLOGICAL TRAUMA

FIGURES

INTRODUCTION

Do your client's families tell them to "get over" their psychological trauma, "move on," or "snap out of it?" But that never seems to work? It doesn't work that way. That's because trauma affects the brain in a way that clients cannot simply "will" themselves out of their symptoms of PTSD or depression. This book, based on our years of research on the brain in PTSD patients, will teach you how to accurately talk to your clients about the body's fear response system and how trauma affects the brain. This can be a highly effective way to formulate the trauma response in a way that is helpful to your clients and their families. This book is aimed at teaching mental health clinicians how to help guide their clients and their partners and families to recovery from psychological trauma.

Psychological trauma can put a stranglehold on your client's life. Childhood abuse, car accidents, sudden death of a loved one, the list is endless. Friends and family may tell them to "get over it," "move on," and "just snap out of it." But it's not that easy. The more they hear things like that, the worse they feel.

Clients can become empowered to take control of their recovery from psychological stress. This book outlines a series of tools you can teach your clients to help them on the road to recovery, including learning about the fear brain, symptoms of traumatic stress, better communication, how medications work, diet and exercise, trauma and the legal system, and more. It can be used in conjunction with *You Can't Just Snap Out Of It: The True Path to Recovery From Psychological Trauma,* which was written for clients affected by psychological trauma.

Guiding Clients in Recovery From Psychological Trauma is specifically focused on providing a guide for mental health workers, including social workers, counselors, therapists, psychologists, and psychiatrists, to help their clients on the road to recovery from psychological trauma. It also provides a useful tool for people working in other fields where they frequently encounter traumatized persons, including legal, pastoral, judicial, and law enforcement. This book comes from the perspective that clients should take charge of their own recovery. Taking charge of their own recovery enhances your client's chances for success. This book will help you teach them how to do that.

CHAPTER 1: PSYCHOLOGICAL TRAUMA: WHAT IS IT AND HOW DOES IT AFFECT PEOPLE?

Psychological trauma, what I have called the "invisible epidemic," is widely pervasive in our society today. Trauma victims suffer from social stigma and negativity from friends and family in their recovery attempts. Comments like "just snap out of it," "move on," and "get over it, move on" are common but not helpful. Often those who claim to be helping may cause more harm than good, either because of a lack of knowledge or because they are linked to the original trauma. Similarly, our legal and law enforcement systems can retraumatize clients, and the slow pace of our court system hinders the recovery process. With so many factors working against them, it's easy for clients to become discouraged. If they don't recover right away, they feel like a failure, which makes recovery even more difficult.

The Scope of Trauma and Its Effects Today

Psychological trauma is defined by the Diagnostic and Statistical Manual (DSM)-5 as a threat to your life or physical integrity or of someone close to you (APA, 2014). Over half of people in the U.S. have been affected by psychological trauma at some time in their lives (Kessler et al., 1995), and this number has increased since the newest version of the DSM (DSM-5) dropped the requirement that the event be experienced with an "intense feeling of fear, horror, or helplessness." Childhood sexual abuse is the most common cause of posttraumatic stress disorder (PTSD) in women. Sixteen percent of women in the U.S. are exposed to sexual abuse at some time in their lives, defined as unwanted sexual contact such as rape or fondling.

The most common cause of PTSD in men is assault. There are a much larger number of civilians in this country with PTSD than former combat veterans suffering with PTSD.

Psychological trauma is associated with a range of adverse physical and health outcomes. These include PTSD and depression, dissociative and anxiety disorders, alcohol and substance abuse, and loss of work productivity. Trauma victims, especially those with PTSD and depression, also use more health resources and have increased rates of heart disease, asthma, and other physical health problems.

Providing Safety

The first step in recovery from psychological trauma is creating a safe environment. Trauma victims cannot begin to recover if they are not in a safe environment. That means that children must be removed from the home of abusers, and threats of violence need to be removed. The perpetrator of violence and abuse should be prosecuted and put in jail, which may give some degree of comfort to the victim. A veteran with PTSD cannot begin recovery until they return from the combat zone. They still need their "combat mind," or heightened fight-or-flight response (which will be discussed in more detail later), in order to survive.

I call the process of moving to a safe place "Coming Home." The meaning of that term is obvious for combat veterans, but I think it is equally applicable to those affected by other types of traumas. A child removed from an abusive home and placed with a supportive parental figure is also "Coming Home." In this context home is wherever a person is safe. Sometimes Coming Home may not occur until someone grows up and establishes a relationship with a supportive partner.

Psychological Trauma is a Disease

The effects of psychological trauma are real disorders, not manifestations of a poor attitude, or moral weakness. I don't have to tell you that as a mental health clinician working on the front lines with victims of psychological trauma, but you may need to convince your clients and their friends and families of this. Psychological trauma-related mental disorders are diseases. Just like for diabetes or heart disease, your clients cannot simply "will" themselves out of the effects of psychological trauma. That is where the mental health profession comes in. Our clients need our help guiding them to recovery.

After a traumatic event, traumatized persons often try to put it behind them, put it out of their minds, forget about it. But unfortunately the trauma has a mind of its own, so to speak. It keeps jumping back into consciousness, sometimes when you'd least expect it. Patients are kept in an endless loop of replaying the memory of the events over and over.

Traumatized people try to think their way out of their disease. But could you think your way out of diabetes? Or heart disease? No way. Why should be it any different for psychological trauma? It's not any different.

It's not uncommon for trauma survivors to put on "a brave face," or a false persona, to cover up the trauma. They look okay on the outside, but inside they are frozen in time, stuck in the grief related to their trauma. They may become super-achievers in an attempt to distract themselves from memories of the trauma or to cover up the feelings of inadequacy and shame that unfortunately are invariably associated with trauma, even when the victims are not to blame. They try to avoid the memories and the pain, through work, or less adaptively through alcohol or drugs, or the distraction of an affairs. Eventually the music stops and they fall off the chair. That's when they find themselves in front of you, the clinician.

Sometimes the suppressed trauma comes out in other ways. Even though the mind suppresses the trauma, it's still there in the body, and the body expresses it through something like a gastric ulcer or a heart attack. Other times it comes out suddenly in the form of a flashback.

I remember when I first recognized the effects of psychological trauma as a physical disease. Many years ago (more than I would like to admit) I was on call as a young psychiatry resident at the Veterans hospital in West Haven, Connecticut. I was woken up from sleep in my on call room by a veteran who had called the operator looking for the psychiatrist on call.

I'd just managed to fall into a fitful sleep when the ring of the telephone pulled me back into the world of the living. The operator patched through a veteran who wanted to talk to the psychiatrist on call.

"Gotta get them out, gotta get them out," the voice on the other end of the line said.

"Excuse me, may I ask who is calling?"

"Gotta get them out, gotta get them out," he repeated in a robotic fashion.

"Who are you, where are you calling from?"

"Gotta get them out. Gotta get them out."

"In order for me to help you, you've got to tell me who you are and what happened tonight."

"Gotta get them out. Gotta get them out."

This went on for twenty minutes. After a while, I talked him down and found out what was going on.

Earlier that night, the veteran rushed into a burning house to rescue three little children. He saved their lives. He was a hero.

But his mind paid a terrible price.

In the Vietnam War, he'd served as a fireman. His job was to put out fires on helicopters hit by enemy fires, including

16

removing people from the flaming aircraft. Sometimes this meant saving lives; other times, it involved just pulling charred bodies out of the wreckage.

His actions as the hero who pulled the three children safely out of the house triggered a flashback to his memories of Vietnam. All he could see, like a movie playing out before him over and over, was a memory from Vietnam, rushing into a burning helicopter and pulling out the charred remains of a twenty-two-year-old marine.

As a last resort, he called the psychiatrist on duty at the VA hospital. Even as he talked to me on the phone, he replayed over and over, like a skip on a vinyl record, or like a continuous computer loop, pulling that body out of the helicopter.

This experience, which I have written about in other books, changed my thinking from a skeptical psychiatric trainee, who wasn't really sure whether these symptoms reported by Vietnam veterans were "real," (an attitude that was unfortunately shared by most mental health professionals at the time), to someone who looked at trauma as a physical disease. This patient reminded me of patients I had treated for epilepsy that originated from the temporal lobe of the brain. Like my patients in the midst of a seizure, he was talking and acting like someone who was awake, but it was not possible to communicate with him.

I wondered if the same part of the brain affected in my epilepsy patients was also responsible for this veteran's behavior? I knew that damage to a specific part of the temporal lobe of the brain called the hippocampus was the origin of my patients' seizures. Neurons in this brain area would start firing rapidly, leading to a seizure. These patients often had feelings of deja vue, or experienced things in a distorted way, much like PTSD patients described the experience of a flashback. I also knew that these symptoms could be recreated by

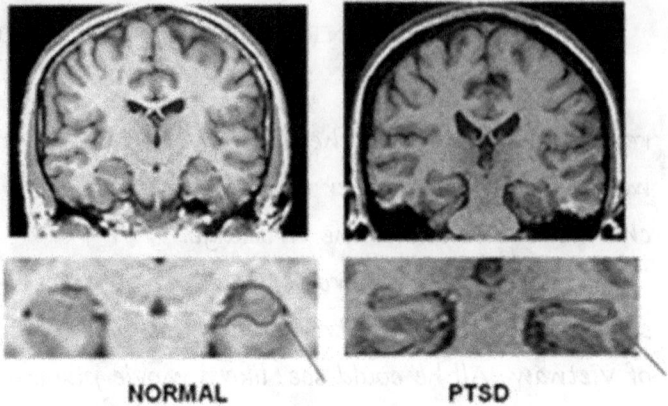

NORMAL　　　　　**PTSD**

FIGURE 1 HIPPOCAMPAL VOLUME IN PTSD

Measured with magnetic resonance imaging (MRI). There is a visible reduction in volume of the hippocampus (outlined in red) in a representative patient with PTSD relative to a normal individual (arrow). Used by permission..

electrically stimulating this part of the brain. Epilepsy patients also have problems with short-term memory, and the hippocampus is known to play an important role in memory.

About this time research was showing that the hippocampus, in addition to being involved in episode, was very sensitive to stress. A scientist from Stanford University named Dr. Robert Sapolsky found that animals exposed to high levels of stress had damage to the hippocampus (Sapolsky, 2004). This led us to wonder whether something similar was going on in our PTSD patients. Using magnetic resonance imaging (MRI), we did brain scans of our patients and compared than to normal subjects without PTSD. We used the MRI scans to measure the volumes of the hippocampi, and found that the PTSD patients had smaller volumes, consistent with a stress-induced effect. We also used neuropsychological testing to show that their ability to remember things, like facts and lists of words, was impaired. These tests included the Wechsler Memory Test, which tests that ability to remember a paragraph, and the Selective Reminding Test, which measures ability to learn a list of words and retain that memory over time. These tests, which are abnormal in patients with hippocampal damage, were also consistent with hippocampal damage.

CHAPTER 2: THE TRAUMA SPECTRUM DISORDERS

The fact that psychological trauma affects mental health has been recognized for the past two centuries, however most of the research on these effects occurred in the last couple of decades.

A History of Diagnostic Approaches to Psychological Trauma

PTSD and the effects of psychological trauma have received more attention over the past few decades than in the past. However we can trace the recognition of what would today be called PTSD back to England in 1830.

The setting was the industrial revolution, when droves of people left their farms, ploughs, and small villages, and headed for the cities to work in factories or other areas of industry. Instead of hobbling along on a horse from village to village, people could now be hurtled across the country in gigantic new contraptions called trains.

Getting all that speed unfortunately brought some dangers. Sometimes the trains crashed into each other or ran off the tracks. Suddenly you had a big accident that involved hundreds of people. These accidents were associated with deaths and injuries.

Doctors started to notice that many of the victims of railroad accidents had persistent symptoms in spite of the fact that they had no identifiable physical injury. This led to the description of what was called "railway spine" in England. A doctor named John Eric Erichsen described the syndrome in 1867 in a book called *On Railway and Other Injuries of the Central Nervous System* (Erichsen, 1867; also see Kirmayer, Lemelson & Barad, 2007). Railway Spine developed in the aftermath of train accidents. It involved symptoms of amnesia,

19

problems with memory, back pain, confusion, and increased anxiety, with no identifiable physical pathology.

Railway Spine was thought to be related to contusions of the spine, which were below the ability of pathological diagnosis to detect. Some authors postulated that Railway Spine could occur in the absence of physical changes. This represented the first description of an effect on the individual of a psychological trauma in which there was not actually a physical injury.

The symptoms of Railway Spine are of course similar to the symptoms of what we today call PTSD. Other symptoms of Railway Spine, like back pain and headache, are commonly associated with PTSD, even if they are not required for the diagnosis.

About that time a German psychiatrist named Oppenheim first described a syndrome he called traumatic neurosis, a disorder in which a traumatic event leads to long-term symptoms. Oppenheim conceived of traumatic neurosis as coming from a psychological stress or shock that lead to long-term changes in physiology. He didn't require an actual physical injury, such as being hit in the head, for the stress to lead to physiological changes in the brain.

The First World War in 1914-1918 was associated with a large number of psychiatric casualties. Doctors in Germany, Italy, and England, described the syndrome of shell shock, in which soldiers would forget their name or where they were on the battlefield. Psychiatrists were tasked with keeping soldiers on the battlefield, which led to increased focus on the syndrome that was impairing the ability of soldiers to be effective in combat. Initially thought to be due to the shock of exploding shells, it was later realized that shell shock could occur even when soldiers were far from an exploding shell. Some authors thought that the psychological trauma itself could be responsible for the symptoms of shell shock.

Around that time the psychoanalytic theory of Sigmund Freud was becoming more prominent. Freud applied his theory of mental symptoms resulting from the suppression of impulses or forbidden desires to the psychiatric casualties. He wrote that a suppressed desire to run from the battlefield explained the symptoms of what he called a traumatic neurosis. Psychoanalysis essentially removed traumatic events or other environmental occurrences from the etiology of psychiatric disorders, relegating them to the products of a purely intrapsychic conflict. The end of the Great War meant that traumatic neuroses were no longer front and center, and interest in this area flagged until the advent of the Second World War in 1941-1945.

Psychoanalysis grew to dominate U.S. departments of psychiatry after WWI. When psychoanalysis was introduced to America, the people who pulled the strings set it up so that only psychiatrists could become trained as psychoanalysts. Training in a psychiatry residency was followed by psychoanalytic training, which involved many years of analysis and supervision. This hopefully led to certification as a psychoanalyst, and was essentially required to get ahead in academic psychiatry. Department chairs in psychiatry were all psychoanalysts. And they controlled psychiatric classifications, which were based on the psychoanalytic theories of Freud. The classification was based on the model that psychiatric symptoms were the result of impulses or desires that were suppressed and unconscious, and that erupted in the form of symptoms.

With the advent of new methods in neuroscience, imaging and genetics, the younger generation of psychiatrists decided that it was time for psychiatry to become more like other disciplines of medicine. That meant it was time to throw out theoretical frameworks for psychiatric diagnosis, and base things on science. Soon the psychoanalysts were thrown out of academic psychiatry, replaced by the new generation of Biological Psychiatrists.

Biological psychiatry laid the foundations for a physical role in the development of symptoms related to emotional trauma. Initially, the focus was on Schizophrenia as a "real" disorder, and the anxiety disorders were left to the psychoanalysts. This led to a persistence of the use of the term "neurosis" in diagnosis, in the form of the "anxiety neurosis."

Veterans returning from the Vietnam War in the 1970s lobbied for recognition of the psychiatric consequences of combat. This led to the description of a Vietnam War syndrome. Authors in the field debated whether these symptoms were a direct result of combat, or related to preexisting personality problems. More research showed that level of combat exposure correlated with symptoms severity, suggesting that the stress of combat itself was responsible for the syndrome (Keane, Caddell, & Taylor, 1988; Keane, Wolfe, & Taylor, 1987).

With the advent of DSM-III, the neuroses were written out of the psychiatric nomenclature and replaced with specific mood and anxiety disorders, including PTSD. The inclusion of PTSD in the DSM-III in 1980 represented the first time that psychological trauma was clearly recognized as playing a central role in the development of a psychiatric disorder.

The Faustian Bargain of DSM-III

I have written before about what I call the "Faustian Bargain" of DSM (see my chapter in Kirmayer, Lemelson & Barad, 2007). Dr. Faust was of course a man who sold his soul to the Devil in exchange for special powers. DSM-III permitted more research and recognition in the field of traumatic stress by creating consistent psychiatric diagnoses. The authors of DSM-III threw out the idea of theoretical constructs, such as psychoanalysis, underpinning psychiatric diagnosis in favor of focusing on the symptoms themselves.

The DSM took at face value presenting symptoms. In cases where symptoms overlapped, they were reworded to appear unique to the disorder. For example, the flat affect of depression is really just another way of describing the experience of feeling cut off or emotionally numb in PTSD. The dissociative experiences of a patient with Dissociative Identify Disorder (DID) were similar to the "flashbacks," of PTSD. Flashbacks are experienced in a dissociated state, complete with feelings of being unreal or in a dream, and are not unique to combat veterans.

Trauma Spectrum Disorders Defined

In my book *Does Stress Damage the Brain?* (WW Norton, 2002) I outlined a group of psychiatric disorders linked to trauma that I argued should be considered part of a spectrum. These disorders, which I termed "Trauma Spectrum Disorders," include PTSD, some cases of depression related to childhood abuse, dissociative disorders (including Dissociative Identity Disorder, or DID), borderline personality disorder (BPD), and some cases of substance abuse and somatization disorders.

As I mentioned above, in 2002 at the time I wrote that book psychiatric diagnosis was based on symptom presentation only. PTSD was grouped in the anxiety disorders only on the basis that it shared with those disorders the clinical presentation of anxiety, even though the source of anxiety in these disparate disorders was likely very different.

Based on the close relationship among dissociation, PTSD and trauma, in *Does Stress Damage the Brain?* I argued for a reorganization of the diagnostic criteria for the anxiety disorders, which in 2002 included PTSD, and dissociative disorders. PTSD doesn't really show much in common in terms of biological changes in the brain with the other anxiety disorders, like obsessive-compulsive disorder (OCD), social phobia, generalized anxiety disorder (GAD) and panic disorder. I argued that PTSD should not be classified as an anxiety disorder, but should rather be included in a group of psychiatric disorders I termed "Trauma Spectrum Disorders." These would include PTSD, BPD, dissociative disorders, and cases of childhood abuse-related depression.

The strengths of a model to describe certain phenomena can be evaluated by its ability to correctly make predictions and to adequately explain the phenomena as they actually occur. The Trauma Spectrum Disorders model was based on the idea that a common neurobiological response to stress underlay these disorders.

We used brain imaging and other measures of neurobiology to test the Trauma Spectrum Disorder model. If the model was correct, we hypothesized that we should see common stress-related changes in the brain, specifically smaller hippocampal volume, a brain area that as reviewed above is known to be sensitive to stress. Disorders outside of the spectrum would be driven by a different neurobiology. For instance, OCD is conceptualized as being due to altered striatal-prefrontal circuits. In fact, in a series of studies, we showed that patients with a history of early abuse and PTSD, DID, depression, and

BPD all shared in common smaller hippocampal volume measured with MRI. This was not seen in patients with panic disorder, or in women with depression without a history of childhood abuse. Other groups showed that OCD and GAD are not associated with smaller hippocampal volume. These studies supported the Trauma Spectrum Disorders model.

Another advantage of the Trauma Spectrum Model was its ability to describe the phenomena of mental disorders as they actually present in clinical practice. Previously psychiatry had been influenced by a desire to be seen as on the same par as other medical specialties. According to this logic, depression is a disease in the same way that diabetes is, caused by a specific defect (the inability of the body to make insulin) and treated with a specific remedy (insulin injections). Likewise, depression was seen as a deficiency of the neurotransmitter serotonin, and the treatment was to "boost" serotonin with serotonin reuptake inhibitor (SSRI) antidepressant medications. Psychiatry as a medical discipline went hand in hand with the development of the psychiatric diagnostic classification system of the DSM-III.

One of the primary theses of the biological psychiatrists was the serotonin model of depression. According to this model, depression was caused by a deficiency of serotonin, which could easily be fixed by drugs that block reuptake of serotonin in the synapse (the Selective Serotonin Reuptake Inhibitors, or SSRIs). The biological psychiatrists became best buddies with the pharmaceutical companies based on their serotonin model, which made for some nifty diagrams in their marketing brochures that they made to sell their exorbitantly priced SSRI drugs, which were still on patent. The patients were told that their depression was not the result of a failure of will or poor life choices, but a chemical deficiency in the brain, so everybody was happy.

The serotonin hypothesis was great for selling drugs, and provided an easy way for patients to think of what was happening to them and how their treatments were working. The only problem with it was that it wasn't true. Neuroscientists and neuropsychopharmacologists have long known that a simple boosting of serotonin could not explain the effects of SSRIs on depression. For one thing, if the hypothesis were true, they should start working right away, and not after 3-4 weeks as they have been shown to in clinical trials.

Besides not being true the serotonin hypothesis had other disadvantages. It was an attempt to bring psychiatry under the "medical model" that governed other medical disciplines. The psychiatrists wanted to be one of the boys (or girls), like their colleagues in cardiology and endocrinology.

The medical model required psychiatric disorders to be discrete entities. You either have diabetes or you don't and there is no overlap with another disorder like cancer, for example. In the same way, it was thought that disorders like PTSD and depression should be discrete and non-overlapping disorders. That led to a lot of problems for those of us in the research world when reviewers of our papers asked us questions like "how do you know that your findings are not due to co-morbid depression." The problem was that they started with the medical model assumption that the two disorders had nothing to do with each other, something that does not fit reality. This caused most clinicians to ignore the diagnostic system developed in the DSM, and to focus on the clinical presentations they were actually seeing in their patients.'

The Trauma Spectrum Disorders model does not assume that these disorders are discrete disorders. It assumes that there are a range of symptoms originating from the body's fear response system that have both overlaps and differences. Many of the symptoms of one disorder can in fact be re-phrased as being the same as symptoms in another disorder, or as being frequently seen in patients diagnosed with that disorder. For instance, the intrusive memories of PTSD can be seen as the ruminations of depression, or the feeling cut off from others or emotionally numb of PTSD is similar to the anhedonia of depression. Thus, the Trauma Spectrum Disorders model is better at explaining the phenomena actually seen in clinical practice, and therefore is more robust than the medical model, and more useful.

Foreshortened future
(suicidality)

Avoidance

Alcohol/substance abuse
*(self destructiveness)*Panic

Decreased
Concentration   Sleep disturbance

Somatization

Hyperarousal,
hypervigilance Feeling cut off   Startle
(agitation)   *(flat affect)*

Flashbacks
*(depersonalization,
derealization)*

Numbing
(anhedonia) Intrusive memories   Amnesia
            (ruminations)   Nightmares

Feeling worse
with reminders
*(Depressed   Decreased
mood)*   interest

Identity disturbance
(dissociative identity d.o.)

PTSD

Brain
Damage

Dissociative
Disorders

Personality
Disorders

depression

Genetics,
prior stressors

Stress

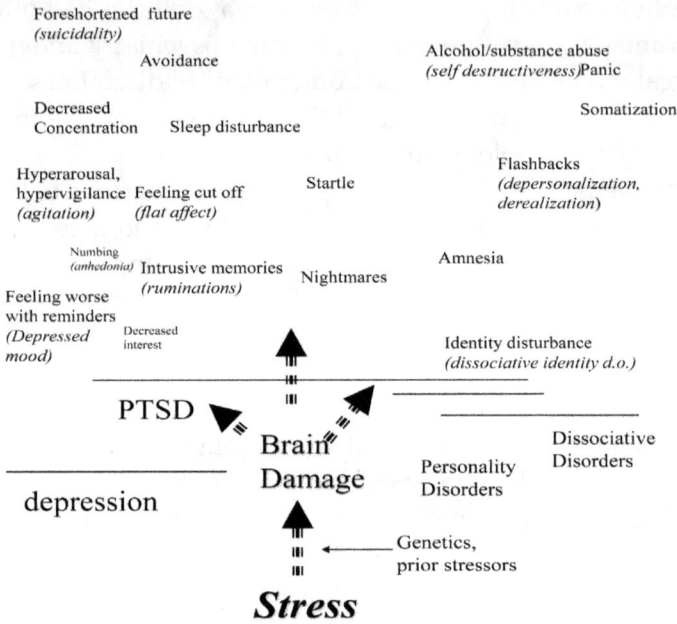

FIGURE 2: TRAUMA SPECTRUM DISORDERS

Trauma leads to a range of symptoms and the symptoms of trauma-related mental disorders often overlap with each other. For instance, in the diagram above, everything the line over "depression" are symptomsm of depression, those above the line over "PTSD" are symptoms of PTSD. As can be seen, the PTSD symptom of feeling cut off from others can be reframed as the depression symptom of flat affect, and so on. This demonstrates that trauma-related mental disorders are not discrete disorders, but rather a spectrum of symptoms with some traumatized persons exhibiting more of one core of symptoms than another. Adapted from figure in *Does Stress Damage the Brain?* (see Appendix C for permissions).

The DSM-5 has since revised the classifications of these disorders. This was probably done in part related to a greater understanding of the neurobiology of these disorders. The Trauma Spectrum Disorders are reviewed in more detail below.

Major Depression

Major depression affects 15% of people at some time in their lives (Kessler, R.C., 2003, JAMA – see Bibliography in Appendix D). Thirty one billion dollars of productivity are lost related to depression in the United States every year (WF Stewart et al, 2003, JAMA). There is more to lost productivity than not showing up for work. Most of it is due to the fact that depressed people spend on average three hours a day doing nothing because they are too depressed. Less than a third of depressed patients, however, are being treated for their depression.

Symptoms of Major Depression

The diagnosis of major depression is based on symptoms of feeling depressed most of the day, every day, for an extended period of time. This is associated with trouble concentrating or focusing, thoughts that the person would be better off dead, or active plans to commit suicide. This may be accompanied by a loss of energy, appetite, and interest in things, decreased interest in sex, loss of pleasure in activities one used to enjoy, and not wanting to be around other people.

Depression is also associated with problems with memory and sleeping, and feeling hopeless and worthless. Depressed patients may have crying spells for no reason, or feel like life is not worth living. Often symptoms of depression appear on the surface to be just relationship problems or difficulty with work or other areas, but the problems are in fact driven by the symptoms of depression.

Depression tends to color the world view of affected patients, changing their perceptions of everything.

DSM CRITERIA FOR MAJOR DEPRESSION
A. At least five of the following symptoms have been present during the same two-week period, and represent a change from previous functioning (one of the symptoms is either a depressed mood or loss of interest or pleasure):
1. Depressed mood most of the day, nearly every day, as indicated either by subjective reports (e.g., feels sad or empty) or observations made by others (e.g., appears tearful)
2. Markedly diminished interest or pleasure in all, or almost all, activities most of the day, nearly every day (as indicated either by subjective account or observations made by others)
3. Significant weight loss when not dieting or weight gain (e.g., a change of more than 5% of body weight in a month), or decrease or increase in appetite nearly every day
4. Insomnia or hypersomnia nearly every day
5. Psychomotor agitation or retardation nearly every day (observable by others, not merely subjective feelings of restlessness or being slowed down)
6. Fatigue or loss of energy nearly every day
7. Feelings of worthlessness or excessive or inappropriate guilt (which may be delusional) nearly every day (not merely self-reproach or guilt about being sick)
8. Diminished ability to think or concentrate, or indecisiveness, nearly every day (either by subjective accounts or as observed by others)
9. Recurrent thoughts of death (not just fear of dying), recurrent suicidal ideation without a specific plan, or a suicide attempt or specific plan for committing suicide.

B. The symptoms do not meet the criteria for a mixed episode (i.e., with manic symptoms included).
C. The symptoms cause clinically significant distress or impairment in social, occupational, or other important areas of functioning.
D. The symptoms are not due to the direct physiological effects of a substance (e.g., a drug of abuse, a medication) or a general medical condition.
E. The symptoms are not better accounted for by bereavement, i.e., after the loss of a loved one, the symptoms persist for longer than two months or are characterized by marked functional impairment, morbid preoccupation with worthlessness, suicidal ideation, psychotic symptoms, or psychomotor retardation.

FIGURE 3: DSM CRITERIA FOR MAJOR DEPRESSION

Post-traumatic Stress Disorder

Another possible consequence of psychological trauma is post-traumatic stress disorder (PTSD).

When we first started our inpatient treatment unit for PTSD at the West Haven, CT, Veterans Administration Hospital, back in 1988, the U.S. Congress awarded us a grant to establish the National Center for PTSD. Our site was the neuroscience research division.

As reviewed above, PTSD was first established as a psychiatric diagnosis in 1980; before that time the medical profession did not recognize that stressful or traumatic events could lead to a psychiatric disorder. We thought that if you had symptoms like PTSD, they were probably related to some other cause—like a bad personality.

This approach is obviously wrong-headed, and not helpful. We have come a long way since that time, but in 1988, most psychiatrists didn't believe in or use the diagnosis of PTSD.

We performed a review of the medical charts at the VA Hospital, and found that none of the patients in our treatment program had ever been diagnosed or treated for PTSD. Their histories were that they came to the VA maybe once in the twenty years after the war, were misdiagnosed as having schizophrenia or some other malady unrelated to the combat experiences, got frustrated, and went back to wherever they came from.

Now we literally had people coming out of the woods, people who had lived in trailers in the remote corners of rural Connecticut with no running water or electricity. When they heard about the availability of a specific treatment for their complaints, they sought it out.

We know a lot more about PTSD today than we did in 1988. That is because we have had more focused treatments, but also because of the research we've performed.

- More than half of Americans will experience a traumatic event at some time in their lives.

- For women the most common type of trauma is sexual abuse or assault, and for men it is physical assault.

- 30% of combat veterans from the Vietnam War
developed PTSD within the first few months of the war,
and it became chronic in 15%.

- These statistics are pretty standard for all types of
trauma, and in men and women.

- 8% of all Americans have PTSD at some time in their
lives, and for reasons that are unclear, it is twice as
common in women as it is in men (Kessler RC, Arch Gen
Psychiatry, 2005).

A history of prior trauma predisposes you to do worse in terms of
PTSD. If you were abused as a child, a rape is more likely to lead to
PTSD. Similarly, in a study we published in *The American Journal of
Psychiatry* in 1993, we found that veterans abused as children were
four times more likely to develop PTSD in Vietnam, even if they were
totally normal when they went overseas.

Not all people exposed to the same level of trauma develop
PTSD, although there is a clear relationship between severity and
repetition of trauma and risk of developing PTSD. I usually tell people
that it is like the relationship between radiation and the risk of
developing cancer; the greater your radiation exposure over the
course of your life, the greater your risk of developing cancer.
However given any two people with the same level of radiation
exposure, one person may develop cancer while the other does not.
This difference may be related to genetics and other factors that we
don't understand.

Post-traumatic stress disorder (PTSD) is by definition linked to a
traumatic event. You also need a minimum number of symptoms
from a Chinese menu.

There are three groups of symptoms of PTSD; namely, intrusions,
avoidance, and hyper arousal. The diagnosis requires one symptom
from the first group, three from the second, and two from the third, as
well as a significant impairment in work and/or social function. These

symptoms come as a result of exposure to an event that is a threat to life of self integrity of yourself or someone close to you.

PTSD intrusive symptoms include recurrent memories of the traumatic event that the individual cannot control, nightmares, feeling worse with reminders, increased physiological responding to reminders (increased heart rate and blood pressure) or feeling as if the traumatic event were recurring.

Many Iraq veterans have increased physiological responding and anxiety when they see something benign like a bag of garbage by the side of the road because this reminds them of Intermittent Explosive Devices (IEDs) often hidden in bags of garbage by the side of the road and detonated by insurgents in Iraq when the armored vehicles drove by on patrols. Fear related to IEDs can turn a simple trip to the grocery store into a terrifying experience.

The second group of symptoms of PTSD is avoidance. These include avoiding things that would remind the person of the trauma, or attempts to avoid thinking about the trauma, having trouble remembering an important aspect of the event, or having a decrease in interest in things they used to like to do (like going to the movies or going fishing). Other avoidance symptoms include feeling detached or cut off from others, distortion of cognitions like having a negative view of the world, feeling emotionally numb or cut off from other people, or having a sense of foreshortened future. Avoidance may manifest in PTSD patients feeling uncomfortable in crowds, or leaving the house.

The third group of symptoms is hyper-arousal. Symptoms of hyper-arousal include trouble falling or staying asleep, increased startle, hypervigilance, irritability, outbursts of anger, reckless or destructive behavior, and difficulty concentrating.

The most recent description of the symptoms is in the DSM-5, which dropped the requirement that the traumatic event be experiences with feelings of fear, helplessness, or horror (American Psychiatric Association, 2013). With this new definition, pretty much the entire population of the U.S. has been exposed to a psychological trauma.

Trauma is Trauma is Trauma

Conceptions of psychological trauma have changed and evolved over the years. Initially we thought of "combat trauma" as distinct from "rape trauma," Holocaust syndrome, childhood abuse, battered woman's syndrome, or other types of traumas. Different countries thought that their own syndromes were unique. For instance, England had "Falkland Islands War Trauma." In the Netherlands, it was "Indonesian War of Independence", Japan was "Tsunami Survivors", and so on. The Germans as a nation exhibited the PTSD symptom of avoidance or psychological denial. With time, however, it became clear that the outcomes of trauma were similar regardless of the type. The only thing that seemed to matter was the age at which the trauma first occurred.

2. Recurrent distressing dreams of the event.

3. Acting or feeling as if the traumatic event were r‹ sense of reliving the experience, illusions, hallucinations flashback episodes, including those that occur on awake intoxicated). Note: In young children, trauma-specific re

4. Intense psychological distress at exposure to inte that symbolize or resemble an aspect of the traumatic ev

5. Physiological reactivity on exposure to internal c symbolize or resemble an aspect of the traumatic event.

C. Persistent avoidance of stimuli associated with the tr‹ general responsiveness (not present before the trauma), (or more) of the following:

1. Efforts to avoid thoughts, feelings, or conversatic the trauma

2. Efforts to avoid activities, places, or people that ‹ the trauma

3. Inability to recall an important aspect of the trau

4. Markedly diminished interest or participation in

5. Feeling of detachment or estrangement from oth‹

6. Restricted range of affect (e.g., unable to have lo‹

7. Sense of a foreshortened future (e.g., does not ex marriage, children, or a normal life span)

D. Persistent symptoms of increased arousal (not preser as indicated by two (or more) of the following:

1. Difficulty falling or staying asleep

2. Irritability or outbursts of anger

3. Difficulty concentrating

4. Hypervigilance

5. Exaggerated startle response

E. Duration of the disturbance is more than 1 month.

F. The disturbance causes clinically significant distress c social, occupational, or other important areas of functio‹ Specify if: Acute: if duration of symptoms is less than 3 duration of symptoms is 3 months or more, or With del‹ symptoms is at least six months after the stressor.

Other Anxiety Disorders Related to Psychological Trauma

Another potential consequence of exposure to traumatic stress is anxiety and panic disorder. Panic is characterized by episodes of extreme anxiety or panic that come out of the blue and make people feel as though they're going to die or go crazy. Associated symptoms include rapid heart rate, feeling as though you can't breathe, muscle tension, nausea, constricted feeling in the chest or throat, sweating, dizziness, and feeling as if you're out of your body or unreal.

Sometimes people with panic disorder have a fear of having an anxiety reaction in public places, in crowds, or while going over a bridge. This can lead to a fear of leaving the house, called agoraphobia, which literally means fear of the marketplace in Greek. Agoraphobia can be very disabling.

Anxiety Disorder Not Otherwise Specified (NOS) means symptoms of anxiety that are disabling but don't fit into one of the other anxiety disorders. These symptoms can include free-floating anxiety associated with trouble breathing, chest pain, nausea, and stomach discomfort. This is another possible outcome of exposure to psychological trauma.

The Effects of Psychological Trauma That Cannot Be Measured

Psychological trauma has lasting effects on the individual not easily captured in our psychiatric diagnostic categories. These include the effects of trauma on the individual's perception of society, the world, and the meaning of their relationship with the world and with others.

The psychiatric disorder, PTSD, is perhaps unique in representing interplay between psychiatric and neurological disease, and a profound alteration in the individual's existential view of the world and his or her place in it. Trauma victims frequently suffer from "survivor's guilt," the feeling that the individual should not have survived when so many others died.

The bare fact that the person survived when so many others perished adds to the feeling that the world is meaningless and nothing makes sense. Victims believe they do not deserve to "leave all of this behind them" and "get on with their life" when only chance led to their survival while others did not survive. They may feel they have more in common with the dead than the living, and that the living do not understand how they feel. This line of thinking can lead to depression and despair, alienation and ultimately suicide and death.

In the next few chapters, I review other consequences of psychological trauma, including borderline personality disorder (BPD), the dissociative disorders, the functional pain disorders, and somatization disorders. I also review how psychological trauma impacts on physical health.

CHAPTER 3: BORDERLINE PERSONALITY DISORDER AND THE DISSOCIATIVE DISORDERS

Borderline personality disorder (BPD) and the Dissociative Disorders are both mental disorders that are frequently associated with a history of childhood stress. Although BPD is currently grouped with other personality disorders in the DSM, like narcissistic personality disorder and avoidant personality disorder, it is one of the psychiatric disorders that were grouped in the trauma spectrum disorders in the book *Does Stress Damage the Brain?* because of its connection with childhood trauma. Even in people without a clear history of trauma, a careful interview often shows that there is a history of emotional abuse, or something about the parent-child interaction in childhood that likely contributes to the disorder. Dissociative disorders are often linked to a history of severe early childhood physical and/or sexual abuse, and were also grouped in the trauma spectrum disorders.

Borderline Personality Disorder (BPD) Defined

BPD is characterized by an intense fear of abandonment by other persons. This results in an instability of interpersonal relationships because the person with BPD desperately tries to pull other people in their lives closer to them, even if it requires a negative strategy to do so. People with BPD also have problems with self-image, mood swings, and impulsive and self-destructive behavior. BPD starts in early adulthood, and can last for months or years. People often get better with time. No two cases are the same.

BPD patients sometimes cut themselves, often repeatedly, for reasons that are not entirely understood. However, a lot of BPD patients will say things like they wanted to replace their inner psychic pain with a physical pain, or that they have an intense feeling of inner emptiness or an uncomfortable feeling that is so unbearable that the only thing that will break it is to cut themselves. Many BPD patients end up with scars on their arms and legs.

These people can damage themselves in other ways, like reckless driving, reckless spending, wild and uncontrolled sex, drugs or drinking, or binge eating. Life with someone with BPD can be a roller coaster ride; you never know what's going to happen next. That's because people with BPD create dramas as a way to prevent people from abandoning them (even if that's totally unrealistic) or to distract themselves from their intense feelings of inner emptiness:

- They do things like make repeated suicide threats or attempts.

- Their mood can swing all over the place.

- They have outbursts of intense anger and irritability.

- Sometimes they have dissociative symptoms, which are describe later in this chapter.

Relationship Between BPD and Psychological Trauma

The link between Borderline Personality Disorder (BPD) and some form of trauma in childhood is clear. Over half of people with BPD were sexually abused in childhood. The risk of developing BPD is increased five-fold after exposure to childhood trauma. About half of BPD patients also have PTSD, while half of PTSD patients have BPD. When BPD patients also have PTSD, they tend to do worse.

Like PTSD patients, BPD patients with a history of childhood trauma have smaller hippocampal volumes and dysfunction in the frontal cortex. We found that BPD patients with early trauma did not react physiologically to reminders of their childhood trauma, but they had huge reactions when read a hypothetical story about a child being abandoned in a shopping mall. This is amazing biological evidence that their fear of abandonment is real, and is wired in the brain (although not necessarily permanently, as is discussed in later chapters on the recovery process from psychological trauma). This probably comes from something that went wrong in early childhood related to how they form attachments to other people, most importantly the people who took care of them (i.e., Moms and Dads). This could be due to physical or sexual abuse, or more likely emotional abuse, or even just a bad fit between parent and child for whatever reason.

Dissociative Disorders as a Consequence of Psychological Trauma

Another group of psychiatric disorders that are often linked to psychological trauma, usually in early childhood, are the dissociative disorders. Dissociation is defined as a breakdown in memory, identity, and consciousness.

Dissociative symptoms include:

- amnesia—gaps in memory not due to ordinary forgetting;

- depersonalization—out-of-body experiences and other distortions of the sense of one's own body, such as feelings that your arms are like toothpicks or your body is very large;

- derealization—distortions in visual perception, such as seeing things as if they are in a tunnel, things are in black and white or colors are very bright, distortions in time, like the feeling that time stands still or is moving very fast, and

- identity disturbance — fragmentation of the sense of the self.

Current DSM-IV dissociative disorders include Dissociative Identity Disorder (DID), Depersonalization Disorder, Dissociative Amnesia, and Dissociative Disorder not Otherwise Specified (DDNOS) (which includes fugue states and derealization disorders, and is sort of a grab bag term for people with disabling dissociative symptoms that don't really fit into any other group).

The Fragmentation of Personality in Dissociative Identity Disorder

Dissociative Identity Disorder (DID) (originally called multiple personality disorder) is characterized by a number of dissociative symptoms as well as disturbances in normal identity. The identity disturbance of DID is really related to a series of amnestic episodes, which when extreme can lead the patient to feel as though there are multiple facets of themselves that are imperfectly connected with one another. The different personality states are often experienced in a dreamy, dissociative state.

DID was previously termed "multiple personality disorder," remember from popular movies like *The Three Faces of Eve*, but the name was changed by the American Psychiatric Association to emphasize the identity fragmentation that occurs in these people. The name change is also in response to extensive media attention, which has focused on the "either/or" aspect of whether an individual has one personality or more than one.

In my clinical work, I have not found this type of dichotomous thinking to be helpful in treating traumatized patients with identity disturbances. Typically, patients describe identity fragments to which they may have attached a name label, and which may have different levels of development but are not completely formed into distinct personalities in the same way that we would think of normal personality. Some of the identity fragments may be associated with painful memories (e.g., a six-year-old fragment who was sexually abused, is very angry, and carries the feelings of fear and shame), whereas others are protected from these painful memories (a ten-year-old "good girl" who is happy and polite).

The identity fragments in DID patients, however, are all part of the same person. As the psychiatrist Colin Ross MD wrote in his book, *Dissociative Identity Disorder*, ultimately it is not possible to have "multiple personalities." Rather, it is the perception of traumatized patients that they have distinct identity fragments within themselves. These identity fragments may play a role in avoiding painful memories of trauma that can incapacitate the individual in his or her daily life. However, ultimately patients need to come to terms with their painful memories and realize that all of the identity fragments are part of just one person.

People often experience traumatic events in a dissociated state. Later, even minor stressors can make them dissociate, or they may dissociate when something reminds them of the original trauma.

Acute Stress Disorder

Acute Stress Disorder (ASD) replaced acute PTSD, which was part of the DSMIIIR and which described episodes of PTSD that occurred during the first month after trauma (since PTSD required a minimum duration of one month of symptoms).

In addition to requiring the presence of a traumatic event, ASD required three of five dissociative symptoms (numbing, derealization, depersonalization, amnesia, or being "in a daze"); one or more of each of the PTSD re-experiencing, avoidance, and hyper arousal symptoms; and functional disturbance (as in DSM-IV PTSD). Most people with ASD go on to develop PTSD.

Dissociation in Response to Trauma

When people dissociate after trauma it can be a sign that things are not going so well. Our studies showed that Vietnam veterans who dissociated at the time of combat trauma were more likely to develop PTSD later, and continued to have dissociative responses to subsequent stressors (Bremner, J. Douglas et al., American Journal of Psychiatry, 1992).

We found that Vietnam combat veterans with PTSD had increased dissociative symptom levels compared to combat veterans without PTSD:

- 86% of patients in a group of Vietnam veterans with PTSD in an inpatient treatment program had the diagnosis of a dissociative disorder, whereas

- Essentially 100% of patients with dissociative identity disorder (DID) in a different inpatient program had a history of severe childhood abuse and the diagnosis of PTSD.

To conduct studies of treatment and neurobiology of dissociation, we developed a scale for use as a repeated measure of dissociative states (mentioned above): the Clinician Administered Dissociative States Scale (CADSS).

The CADSS is a nineteen-item scale administered by a clinician who begins each question with the phrase "at this time" and then reads the item to the subject. The subject then endorses one of a range of possible responses: 0 not at all, 1 slightly, 2 moderately, 3 considerably, 4 extremely.

Some of the dissociative symptoms measured with the CADSS that were most commonly endorsed in traumatized patients included

- "Did things seem to be moving in slow motion?"

- "Did sounds change, so that that they became very soft or very loud?" and

- "Did it seem as if you were looking at things as an observer or a spectator?"

We found that these symptoms increased when PTSD patients were re-exposed to reminders of their original trauma during a traumatic memories group I conducted at the inpatient PTSD program at the VA hospital.

Dissociation and Psychosis

Sometimes dissociative symptoms can resemble symptoms of psychosis, like seeing things that are not there or hearing voices, even the perception of the voice of a dead person whom the victim of psychological trauma once knew.

Dissociation, however, is usually related to a traumatic event, whereas psychotic symptomatology does not show such a specific connection with trauma.

Psychotic auditory hallucinations, on the other hand, commonly consist of an unrecognized foreign voice with specific types of content, such as making disparaging comments about the individual. Finally, visual hallucinations in dissociative disorders are related to the traumatic memory and involve the perception of normal "intact" scenes, whereas psychotic visual hallucinations have bizarre content and often involve a breakdown of the scenario of the scene.

Dissociation and Trauma: A Case Study

One of the best ways to understand the symptoms of dissociation is to look at the story of someone who is affected by them. In my book *You Can't Just Snap Out Of It* I talked about a patient I had, whom I'll call "Chuck," who was a combat veteran in the Vietnam War. He said that after a fire fight, they moved in to kill off the enemy with bayonets. They stabbed the enemy rather than shooting them so that they would not alert the Viet Cong that they were in the area.

He said, "While we were stabbing the enemy, I felt myself drifting above the scene. I was looking at myself from a distance. That person down there was 'a Killer,' but it really wasn't me. I felt sorry for him."

This is an example of depersonalization, i.e., when you see things from outside of yourself. Other people feel distortions in their body — their arms are like toothpicks, or their body becomes very large.

I had another patient I'll call Frank who also had PTSD from Vietnam. He would be sitting on the couch next to his wife having an argument, and another person would pop up next to him, an alternative version of himself. It would be the "fighter" version of himself, ready to knife someone in the gut, or throw machine gun fire into a village without knowing who was in there — things he would not attribute to himself as things that he could easily do. He saw this person as someone different from himself.

One time he was arguing with his wife and this alternative version of himself popped up next to himself and said, "She's a bitch, hit her, she won't know the difference."

Another vet with PTSD, named Harry, used to see his buddies who died in Vietnam sitting in his car while he drove around. One day he was drinking on his back porch and he saw a helicopter landing in his back yard with his dead buddies. He saw them in a dissociated state, as though in a dream, colors were very bright, and time seemed to stand still.

His young daughter said, "Daddy, just let them go."

Later when he was drinking in his basement, they came to him. They told him to kill himself so that he could join them.

Years later, after he had completed our program, I heard that someone had pushed him in front of a subway train in New York. I never learned the details of that event.

Trauma and Development

To understand dissociative identity disorder, it is important to have an understanding of normal personality development. Almost

44

all cases of dissociative identity disorder are related to early childhood abuse.

Childhood abuse can have lasting effects on the sense of self. Our sense of self does not exist from the time of birth; rather, it is the result of an accumulation of a lifetime's experiences and positive relationships with others. For example, a particularly positive experience with a math teacher will allow the individual to "take away" an aspect of that role model's personality, incorporate it into the sense of self, and lead to a strengthening of the personality.

A more fundamental example of this phenomenon is the interaction between infant and mother. This is what Winnicott (1965) and others who wrote about object relations theory called the phenomenon of the "good enough mother."

In abusive families, the mother may not only be not "good enough," but may actually be a source of threat. This has an important impact on the child's development of the sense of self, leading to a fragmentation of identity and a walling-off of aspects of memory and the self.

Childhood abuse can also be associated with lasting feelings of shame (related to a common process of self-blame) and rage against the perpetrator and others in the family who did not protect them. A sense of powerlessness in the face of the abuser can put the abuse victims at risk for becoming perpetrators themselves when they become adults, in an attempt to have the feeling of power over another that they could not have as children.

I talk more about the effects of trauma on the brain and how this interacts with physical health in the next chapter.

CHAPTER 4: EFFECTS OF TRAUMATIC STRESS ON THE BRAIN

Psychological trauma can have long-term effects on the brain that complicate the recovery process. As discussed in the book *Does Stress Damage the Brain? Understanding Trauma-related Disorders from a Mind-Brain Perspective*, changes in the brain after trauma can affect the behavior and emotions of the trauma victim. And it can do this in a way that makes it basically impossible to simply "will" oneself out of the situation.

To understand how psychological trauma affects the brain, we must first understand something about the nature of the brain itself.

Our Mysterious Brains

The brain is the most complicated, but also the most interesting, organ of the body. It is the central clearinghouse of everything that matters to us as individuals.

Prior civilizations considered the heart or the liver to be the center of the personal essence or spirit. The Greeks had a word called "thumos," meaning courage or strength of character. They thought thumos was in the chest somewhere.

People still use phrases like "he has a good heart" or they talk about someone "dying of a broken heart." Some of those old ideas about emotions living in the chest haven't completely gone away.

Today we would put thumos in the brain, and think of it as related to the mind. Now we know that the mind is in the brain. That is why there has been a sudden burst of interest in the field of neuroscience amongst the general public.

People want to learn more about themselves and how they fit into the world. Many people now realize that the brain, rather than being something relegated to dry textbooks, is a thing of mystery and complexity. It is important to understand and celebrate it, something to be embraced as a rich source of knowledge that will help us on our path toward a greater understanding of ourselves.

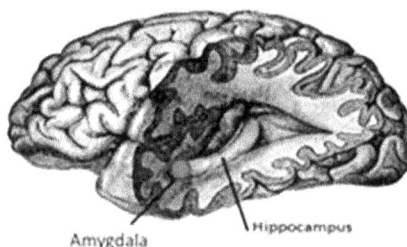

Amygdala   Hippocampus

FIGURE 5: DIAGRAM OF THE HUMAN BRAIN SHOWING THE HIPPOCAMPUS AND AMYGDALA

Diagram of the human brain from the side with a cut-away section showing the hippocampus (colored in blue) and amygdala (colored in red). The frontal lobe (front of the brain) is on the left side of the diagram. The amygdala sits at the head of the hippocampus. There is a hippocampus and amygdala on both the left and the right sides of the brain. (Source: Wikipedia)

Understanding the Brain as Part of the Process of Recovery

Teaching your clients about the brain and fear response systems can be a useful tool in helping them on the road to recovery. Using the language of neuroscience helps objectivity the PTSD experience and takes it away from the idea that PTSD symptoms represent a moral or personal weakness. It can It can also be a way for families to understand what is happening to their loved ones and not blame themselves, or give unhelpful feedback. You're probably already using the language of neuroscience, but if don't have neuroscience training, you might be wondering if your explanations are always accurate. As a researcher specializing in the neuroscience of fear responses in the brain, I will teach you in this chapter what you need to know to effectively and accurately explain the physiological response to trauma and how it manifests itself in symptoms to your clients.

To answer these questions, we have to learn a little bit about how the brain and the physical senses work.

How the Brain Perceives the World

How do things in the world affect us? How do we taste, hear and feel, and how can these things influence our emotions, our sense of self and others?

Studies showed that previously healthy journalists who watched executions of prisoners were often affected for years afterward by mental health problems, even though they didn't personally know the person being executed, even though they were not physically harmed or injured in any way (at least on the outside.) Why is it that passively watching something like an execution can have such a devastating impact on us? Why is it that the witnessing of a terrible event, acting through our vision, hearing, smell, and other senses, can change our lives, possibly forever?

When we smell something, small amounts of substances are emitted from the thing we smell that physically enter our nose and travel through little holes in the top of our nose, in an area called the cribriform plate. They next land on a part of the brain, the olfactory cortex, that is responsible for smell.

Isn't that amazing?

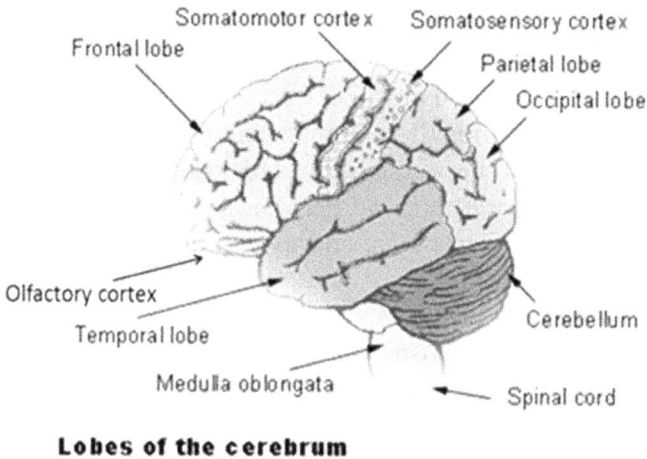

Lobes of the cerebrum

FIGURE 6: VIEW OF THE SURFACE OF THE HUMAN BRAIN

The cerebrum, or cerebral cortex, is at the outer part of the brain, and includes frontal and temporal lobes and other areas. The frontal lobe is involved in thought and emotion and suppression of fear reactions from the amygdala. The olfactory cortex, that processes smell, is in the orbitofrontal cortex at the bottom part of the frontal lobe. The somatomotor cortex controls movement of the body. The somatosensory cortex processes feelings of touch. The visual cortex that processes what we see is in the occipital lobe, which is at the back of the brain. Auditory cortex (sound) is in the temporal lobe. The brain stem, which controls basic processes like breathing or sleep, is the pink area, and includes medulla oblongata and spinal cord. (Source: Wikipedia)

This brain area sends the information on to the rest of the brain. For instance, if you smell rotting meat, invisible pieces of the meat waft in the air (because they are so small they can get blown around easily), travel through your nose, and are detected by the brain as having something wrong with them.

The olfactory cortex then sends a signal to the fear area of the brain, called the *amygdala*, that says, "Danger, danger! We've got rotten meat here that may contain bacteria and kill you if you eat it. I don't care how hungry you are, don't do it!"

The amygdala sounds the alarm, causing hormones like cortisol and norepinephrine to flood the body. This results in increases in heart rate and blood pressure and breathing.

It also causes shifts in where energy is sent to in the body, that may help us survive.

We'll talk in more detail   e body during the fear response.

Different parts of the brain work together to process what's going on in the world. They have to work together as an effective team. If they didn't, we wouldn't survive.

Everything we see, smell, hear, taste and touch gets processed by different parts of the brain. If the brain detects a threat, it activates the fear response. If you walk down a path in the jungle and bump into a lion, a series of things happen in your brain that end up with the thought, "Get the heck out of here!"

The vision of the lion comes in through the eyes and is sent to a part of the brain called the primary visual cortex, or occipital lobe, which is in the very back of the brain. It then goes to the secondary visual association cortex, right next to it, where a more complicated processing of the vision takes place. The lion growls, and the noise comes in through the ears and is sent to the auditory cortex, a part of the brain in the temporal lobe that processes sounds.

The parts of the brain involved in memory, the hippocampus and frontal cortex, pull this information together and compare it to prior experiences of running into a lion. If there's a match, the information is sent to the amygdala, which cranks up your heart rate, blood pressure, and breathing. You brain then tells you "Let's get out of here!" Otherwise, you might become lunch.

The Science of Fear Learning

Specific parts of the brain are involved in learning fear. In experiments with rats where you pair a bright light with a shock, exposure to the light alone will cause a fear reaction. This is called fear acquisition, fear conditioning, or acquisition of conditioned fear. It is called conditioning, because we become "conditioned," or learn to be afraid, in specific situations.

If there is damage to the amygdala, animals don't learn fear reactions. That tells us that we learn fear, or acquire conditioned fear responses, with the amygdala.

The ability to learn fear reactions is very important for survival, absolutely necessary, in fact. If we don't learn fear, we become somebody else's lunch.

PTSD is the Failure to Unlearn Fear

Just as important as learning fear, is the ability to unlearn it. Although not learning fear will make you into lunch, not being able to unlearn it will make you miserable — you might wish you had been lunch.

To get back to our rats, with continued exposure to the light without the shock, the animal will "learn" there is no danger associated with the light, and the fear reaction will go away. This is called "extinction" of fear. It results from the frontal cortex (the part of the brain in the front) sending signals to turn off the amygdala. Animals with damage to the frontal cortex have problems turning off the fear response. PTSD is like a kind of failure to unlearn fear.

A guy named Phineas Gage, who lived about 100 years ago, had a railroad spike go into his frontal cortex and damage that part of the brain. After that, although he had normal speech and seemed OK, he had difficulties regulating his emotions and interacting with other people. This led doctors to the idea that this part of the brain was involved in emotion.

Did you ever get in a car accident? Remember how right after that you were afraid to get behind the wheel again? And that after a while when you kept driving, because otherwise how else would you get to work, the fear reaction went away? That is an example of fear acquisition and extinction. People with PTSD are not able to turn off the fear reaction normally, which is what often makes them disabled.

Sometimes It's Better Not to Go on Vacation

Sigmund Freud, the great Austrian psychoanalyst, said that you have to go on vacation for at least a month to get any benefit out of it. People do that in Europe, where my wife comes from. In fact, everyone goes to the beach for the entire month of August. Although we don't do that in the U.S., everyone agrees that vacation is a good thing.

Actually that isn't always true. I'll tell you why in a minute.

One of the things I love about giving lectures to a new groups of people is that, while I have something to teach them about my knowledge and expertise in psychiatry and neuroscience, they usually have equally useful and information for me. For example, many years ago I gave a lecture about psychological trauma to a group of Navy psychiatrists in Norfolk, Virginia. After the lecture, the psychiatrists talked about some of their patients who were on active duty.

One of the psychiatrists shared a story of an enlisted man in the Navy who was on a submarine that experienced an on-board explosion while out to sea. No one was injured, but the Navy thought they would do him a favor and give him a week of shore leave. It turned out not to be a favor at all.

When he walked out on the dock at the end of his leave time to get back on the sub, he couldn't make himself move. By keeping him away from the source of the accident, they hadn't allowed his normal fear extinction functions to work. His fear became ingrained in his brain, and now it would be harder than ever to get over it. You see, it would have been better if they didn't give him a vacation. I'm not sure if that sailor ever did get back on a submarine.

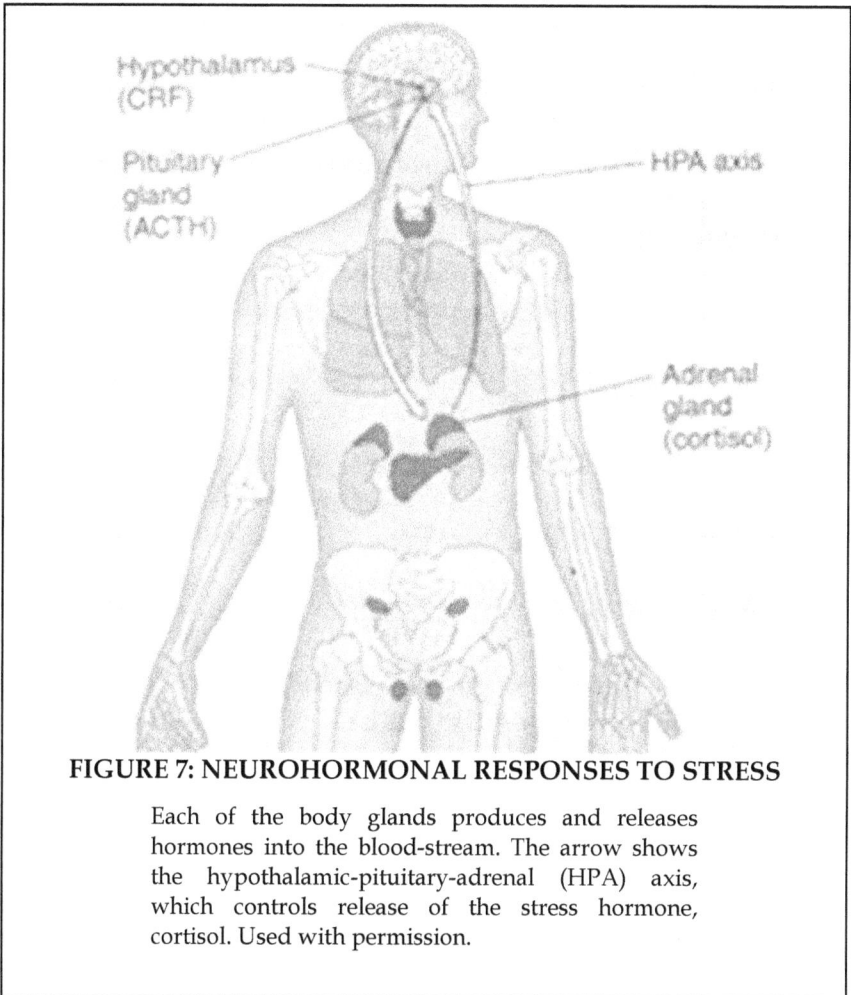

FIGURE 7: NEUROHORMONAL RESPONSES TO STRESS

Each of the body glands produces and releases hormones into the blood-stream. The arrow shows the hypothalamic-pituitary-adrenal (HPA) axis, which controls release of the stress hormone, cortisol. Used with permission.

Stress Hormones and the Fear Response in Survival

Part of team brain response to survival is an outpouring of stress hormones like norepinephrine and cortisol that flood the body during stress. Like the amygdala, they also help us survive. Let's see how they work.

A collection of brain cells (or neurons) in the brain stem (the part of the brain at the back of your neck that controls basic functions like breathing and being awake) contains the majority of the stress hormone, adrenaline, in the brain. Technically, it is known as noradrenaline (norepinephrine) when it occurs in the brain and adrenaline (epinephrine) in the body, but I refer to both using the commonly known term "adrenaline."

These brain cells have long fibers, known as axons, that extend their tentacles throughout the brain, and release adrenaline everywhere all at once. This release is triggered by a scary event, like the attack of a lion. Adrenaline acts like a chemical messenger that says "RUN!!"

Adrenaline is the Brain's Fire Alarm System

When there's a fire, you run and pull an alarm that tells everyone in the building to get out right away. The idea is to tell everyone to leave, both the people who might get burned and those who are not at risk. There will be time to sort that out later, but in the short term it is better to make sure that everyone is safe.

Our brains and bodies have their own fire alarm system. It's called adrenaline. When there's a threat, adrenaline is released everywhere, signals all parts of the brain to pay attention, and triggers all parts of the body to be ready. Adrenaline makes blood pressure go up and heart rate increase so that you can deliver more blood to your brain, muscles, and the other parts of the body important to survival. You breathe faster so you get more oxygen into your lungs and then your blood. More blood means more oxygen and more energy (sugar) to help those body parts work better, so you can run faster and fight harder.

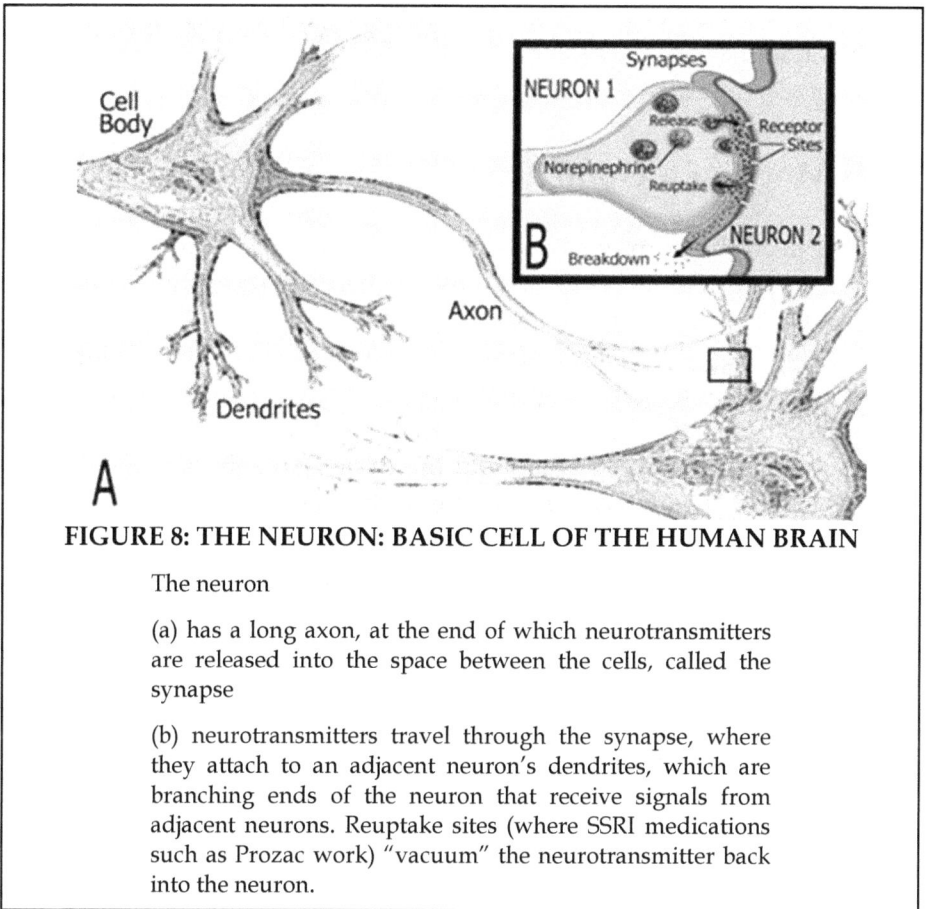

FIGURE 8: THE NEURON: BASIC CELL OF THE HUMAN BRAIN

The neuron

(a) has a long axon, at the end of which neurotransmitters are released into the space between the cells, called the synapse

(b) neurotransmitters travel through the synapse, where they attach to an adjacent neuron's dendrites, which are branching ends of the neuron that receive signals from adjacent neurons. Reuptake sites (where SSRI medications such as Prozac work) "vacuum" the neurotransmitter back into the neuron.

Cortisol Chips In

At the same time that your adrenaline system is firing, corticotropin releasing factor (CRF) is released from a part of the brain called the hypothalamus. This triggers a chain reaction which results in the release of the stress hormone, cortisol, from the adrenal gland.

Cortisol helps to move energy to the muscles so we can fight back or run away fast. It does this by moving energy away from areas that aren't needed for survival, like the stomach (you don't need to digest your lunch right away) or reproductive organs. Fast thinking and strong muscles are critical to survive at that split second when we are under attack.

Too Much of a Good Thing

We need the hormones cortisol and adrenaline to help us survive, but if we are under stress for too long, or there are too many traumatic events, they can get out of whack.

In some cases, CRF and adrenaline can be chronically too high; as well, minor stressors or things that trigger memories of stress may cause you to release way too much cortisol and norepinephrine. The cortisol system may get burnt out, it might not have the right rhythm, or it might be depleted at certain times of the day.

The fear part of the brain, the amygdala, may be over-active, and the parts of the brain involved in memory and emotion and turning off the fear response (the hippocampus and frontal cortex) may not turn on normally. You might use alcohol and drugs to turn off these stress hormones and quiet your brain so that you don't feel so anxious, but that can become a problem in itself. We will talk more about brain areas involved in stress later on.

How Psychological Trauma Affects the Brain: Case Study

I once had a patient who was a successful executive in a manufacturing company who had to travel frequently for business.

One morning, she was staying at a hotel and opened the door to see if the newspaper was there. A homeless man lurked in the hallway eating food off of the trays left out the night before. He pushed his way into her room and assaulted her. He had been drinking coffee off the trays in the hallway so he had coffee on his breath. He pulled on her hair from behind while he attempted to sodomize her. She managed to get away and alert hotel security, who had him arrested.

Following this, her body's fear response system activated when things reminded her of the event, even when no true threat existed. The smell of coffee caused an outpouring of adrenaline in her body, just as it did when she was assaulted. Her heart rate and blood pressure went up, and she started breathing rapidly.

When her three-year-old daughter pulled on her hair while playing, it made her feel extremely anxious and fearful. Her heart raced, and she felt as though she had to get away. This made it difficult for her to spend time with her daughter. She developed other symptoms of PTSD, like being jumpy and easily startled, having nightmares and flashbacks of the event, having trouble sleeping and concentrating, and trying to avoid things that reminded her of the event.

Whereas before she had a job with a lot of responsibility, she now found it difficult to get through the day. She had problems remembering things.

She said, "Lately I feel like my mind is degenerating, like I have some horrible dementing illness, I can't remember anything or think about anything normally. I walk into a room and I see something I've never seen before, and I say to myself, 'I've never seen that before, where did that come from?' I feel like I am falling apart."

When we read back a description of her rape incident to her in the laboratory while measuring her stress hormones, her body flooded with the stress hormone, cortisol, three or four times higher than normal, and her heart rate and blood pressure increased dramatically. We next read a description of the trauma to her while she was lying in a positron emission tomography (PET) camera, which measures brain function. The part of the brain responsible for thinking clearly and putting a brake on anxiety reactions, called the frontal cortex, shut down, as did her hippocampus, a brain area involved in memory. Other brain areas that drive the fear response were put in overdrive.

The Brain Remembers Trauma

Memories for the things that happen to us in daily life are formed by a brain area called the hippocampus, but the hippocampus doesn't store everything in memory forever. Sherlock Holmes's sidekick, Dr. Watson, had a theory about memory he called the Crowded Lumber Room Theory that was actually correct. It you put some wood into a crowded lumber room, you're going to have to take some other wood out to make room for the new wood. It is the same for memory. Store some new memories, take other ones out.

How does the brain do this? It stores the memories for a short time in the hippocampus. After the course of hours or days, some memories get moved into long-term storage in the cerebral cortex. This process is called *memory consolidation*.

But how does the brain decide which memories should be kept and which discarded? Obviously some memories are more important to keep than others. A lion attack is an experience you will probably never forget. That's a good thing, because the next time you see a lion, you be prepared to take appropriate action.

How does your brain keep the memory of the lion and not the memory of what you had for breakfast this morning? When cortisol and adrenaline are released during stress, they act on brain areas like the hippocampus that are involved memory to strengthen the memory trace. These hormones also tie the memory to the actual memories of the emotion, stored in a brain area called the amygdala. That way, the next time you see the lion, your fear response will come back right away, which will then prepare your body to deal with the potential threat.

Effects of Trauma on the Brain

The brain doesn't always respond to trauma in the most efficient way. The flood of stress hormones can cause damage to the hippocampus, the brain area responsible for forming memories. The stress hormones can also make the memory fragmented, dream-like, or distorted in other ways.

Depending on their concentration and how the brain has been affected by psychological trauma, stress hormones may cause traumatized individuals to not remember some things or some parts of the trauma well or not at all. In some cases, the hormonal response to stress is permanently changed, so that whenever there is a reminder of the event (like seeing a lion again), cortisol and adrenaline flood into the brain.

The flooding of these hormones also affects how the memory is recalled. The memory can pop into the mind of your client at all times of the day and night, *so that they can't stop thinking about it* – like when you try to save a document on a computer in the midst of crashing. The document is often stored in a damaged way. As a result, every time you go to turn on the computer, the document pops up onto the screen. *It doesn't wait until you decide to access it.*

When I started out as a researcher in psychiatry, working in an inpatient hospital unit for the treatment of Vietnam veterans with PTSD, we saw a presentation by a famous neuroscientist named Robert Sapolsky, PhD, about the effects of stress on the brain of monkeys.

He found that male monkeys who had been severely stressed by being caged with female monkeys (the females beat up the males in that particular species of monkey) had damage to the part of the brain involved in learning and memory called the hippocampus.

The brain cells, or neurons, showed a loss of the normal branching that under a microscope looks like the branches of a tree –

the stressed monkeys had hippocampal neurons that looked like a withered tree.

Other scientists later found that the hippocampus was unique in the brain, the area where new neurons could be developed in adulthood. Stress unfortunately had the effect of turning off the growth of new neurons.

Smaller Hippocampal Volume in PTSD Patients

We wondered if stress could have a similar effect in our combat veterans, so we used magnetic resonance imaging (MRI) to measure the size of this brain structure in our veterans with PTSD. To our surprise, we found an 8% reduction in volume in this brain area. Later studies showed that people with PTSD from childhood abuse also had a reduction in volume in this area.

When we gave tests of the kind of memory the hippocampus is responsible for — learning new things like what to buy at the grocery store, or remembering the content of a story that was read out loud — they showed significant impairments. Since then many other research groups and scientists have had similar findings in a range of different groups of patients with PTSD.

For instance, when we did an MRI scan of the brain of the woman who had been a rape victim in a hotel that I described above, and measured the size of her hippocampus, we found it to be reduced in size, consistent with a stress-induced shrinkage.

PTSD as a Memory Disorder

We like to think of PTSD as a memory disorder because many PTSD patients have trouble remembering things, like where they have to go or what they have to do that day, while other things, especially their trauma, they can't get out of their minds. That is why we call it the "can't stop thinking about it disease."

While some parts of the trauma come back as repetitive intrusive memories, other important details of the trauma can't be remembered at all. One of the possible consequences of psychological trauma are symptoms of dissociation. These include feelings of being unreal, out of body, gaps in memory, or feeling like you are in a dream or a daze.

Trauma victims with the most severe hippocampal shrinkage have the most trouble with memory and the most dissociative symptoms. These victims have the greatest trouble because the hippocampus is responsible for memory as well as our perception of where we are in time and space (felt to represent a critical aspect of dissociation). We talk about dissociation in more detail later.

The Frontal Cortex Saves the Day (Or Not)

Another brain area that plays an important role in controlling our anxiety and fear reactions is the frontal cortex. This brain area has grown and grown as humans have evolved and is what makes us different from monkeys and all other animals down the line. The growth of this part of the brain allowed us to do all sorts of awesome things like make things, talk to each other, write books like this one, and figure out in our heads whether we have enough money to buy a latte at Starbuck's.

Unfortunately, getting a bigger brain also had its drawbacks. It's because we have this humongous brain area that we spend way too much time worrying about things we don't have any control over, anyway. This part of the brain is also sensitive to stress. Animals exposed to stress early in life have a decrease in branching of the neurons in this part of the brain. If there is something that looks like it might be scary, but isn't really, this brain area shuts off the fear reaction from the amygdala. We found that patients with PTSD, whether it is from childhood trauma or combat trauma, don't activate this part of the brain normally when they are listening to a script of their childhood trauma or watching combat scenes. We think this brain problem is the reason they have fear reactions all the time, even if there isn't something that is a real danger to them.

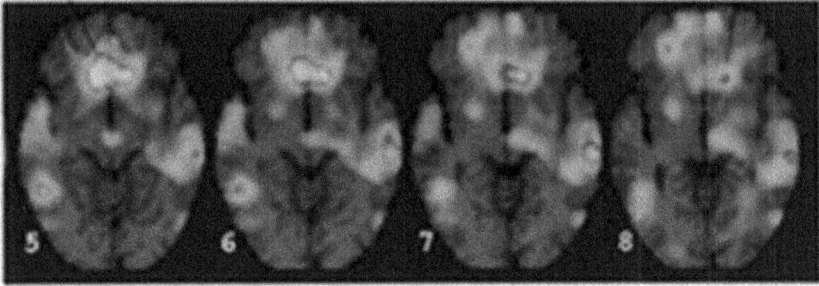

FIGURE 9: EFFECTS OF TRAUMATIC REMINDERS ON BRAIN FUNCTION

Brain activation with exposure to traumatic reminders measured with positron emission tomography (PET) brain imaging. The image shows where there are difference in blood flow in the brain between combat veterans with and without PTSD while viewing combat-related slides and sounds. Combat veterans withà PTSD compared to those without PTSD had a decrease in brain function in the medial prefrontal cortex (PFC) (yellow area), including the anterior cingulate (AC), during exposure to combat-related slides and sounds. Used by permission from J. Douglas Bremner, M.D.

The Stress Response Gone Haywire

With repeated stress and traumas over time, the parts of our body responsible for our survival start to go haywire. The cortisol and adrenaline hormones that help us run away or fight back get out of whack, the hippocampus that helps us remember past threats gets damaged, the amygdala that activates the fear response over-reacts, and the frontal cortex that turns off the fear response doesn't work the way it used to.

This results in a chronic state of anxiety, over-activation of the fear response, a withdrawal from the world in an attempt to deal with our fears, and a general lack of adaptation to the world:

- The soldier who returns from Iraq looks for the switch to turn off his combat reaction, but he doesn't find it because it doesn't exist.

- The woman who was a victim of rape tries to "move on" with her life and start to date men again, but she is overcome with anxiety and fear, and cannot stand to have people get close to her, literally.

These are all situations where PTSD sufferers cannot just will away their responses because the responses are ingrained into their brains and bodily response systems. They can't just "get over it," because it is not in their power to do so.

So what should they do?

How to Start to Move On From Psychological Trauma

The first step on the pathway to recovery from psychological trauma for your clients is to identify the invisible barriers blocking them. I will expand upon this in the next chapter.

You can help educate your traumatized clients about what trauma is and the corrosive and subtle ways it can affect them.   Teach them that it's not their fault for not getting over it. And that recovery from trauma is a process, involving psychotherapy and the others methods outlined in this book.

CHAPTER 5: BARRIERS TO RECOVERY

As I discussed in the last chapter, if not dealt with correctly, trauma leads to changes in the brain that make the painful memories keep coming back when they are least expected. To get rid of these painful memories and the emotions that flood the body, people initiate evasive maneuvers. They drink or take drugs to dampen down the feelings, to eliminate the stress hormone responses and to blot out the painful memories. But these behaviors can become barriers to recovery from psychological trauma.

Research has shown that alcohol and drugs, like heroin, or related pain killers, like oxycodone, sedating benzodiazepine drugs (Xanax, Valium), and marijuana, actually reduce the stress hormones and make stress systems better…in the short term. The problem is that sooner or later these effects go away, and then the trauma victim is left with the stress symptoms again… along with a hangover, and maybe a DUI, addiction, or a pink slip.

Some people may work all the time, or lose themselves in endless affairs, or find other activities to distract their minds from their traumas. These people go to extraordinary ends to avoid their memories, but they are fighting against the tide, because trauma has changed their neurological systems. In effect, they are fighting against their own mind, brain, and body.

All of these ways to try and get away from the trauma are ultimately barriers to recovery.

The Desperate Need to Escape from Trauma

The desire to suppress the memories of the traumatic event can result in long-term harm to the psyche and/or in self-destructive behaviors we use to distance ourselves from the initial trauma.

64

Although this struggle to suppress the traumatic memories is ultimately futile, unfortunately too many well-intentioned people — family, friends, even some professionals — who regularly counsel trauma victims to do just that: try to forget about it, or just get over it.

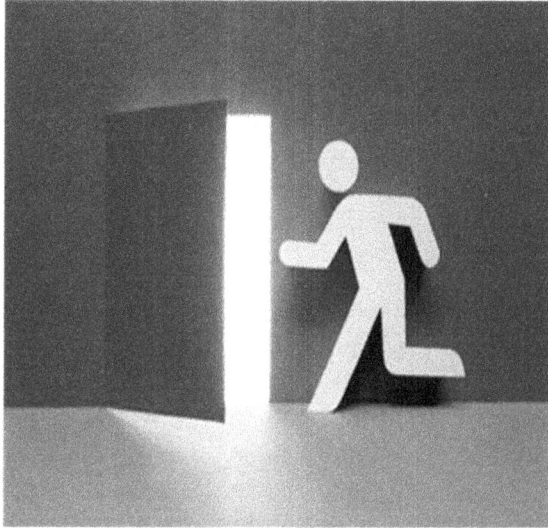

FIGURE 10: THE NEED TO ESCAPE

When well-intentioned people consistently advise trauma victims to forget about their traumatic experiences, those victims can easily fall into depression, substance abuse, self-loathing, or feelings of extreme inadequacy. These responses, a natural by-product for some reason of psychological trauma, are compounded by the feeling of futility and inadequacy that comes with the realization that they can't just "got over it."

Although later it becomes patently obvious that these destructive behaviors are the result of the trauma, at the time, and often for many years afterward, most people do not make the connection for the following reasons:

1. they were so engaged in their futile attempts to flee the memories, they did not stop long enough to ask themselves why they were so self-destructive, and

2. it was suggested — explicitly and implicitly — by a host
   of people that they were doing harmful things, not
   because they had experienced a bad event, but because
   they were bad people.

Many trauma victims fall for this line of thinking. When you are told by an authority, either directly or indirectly, whether that authority is a TV psychologist, or a teacher or a parent, that you are bad, you tend to believe the authority, especially when you get this message as a child. And once you have taken the message in, it's hard to get rid of it.

Self-Medication of Trauma

We worked with scientists at the Centers for Disease Control (CDC), our next door neighbor at Emory University in Atlanta, Georgia, and demonstrated that childhood abuse increases the risk for intravenous drug abuse in adulthood by over TEN TIMES. (It also increases the risk of cigarette smoking.) This is equivalent to the risk of getting lung cancer if you smoke cigarettes. We all know that smoking cigarettes causes lung cancer, but did we know that childhood abuse causes drug addiction?

I don't think so.

In traumatized people, PTSD and alcohol and substance abuse often occur together:

- 80% of Vietnam veterans with PTSD have a history of alcoholism or substance abuse at some time in their lives, more than double the rates seen in veterans without PTSD.

- 28% of American women with PTSD have a history of alcoholism, compared to 14% of women without PTSD (see my book *Does Stress Damage the Brain?* 2002).

Our research showed that PTSD patients abuse alcohol and substances as a form of self-medication (Bremner et al, *American Journal of Psychiatry*, 1996).

Why does trauma cause drug addiction?

You'll remember that the stress hormone adrenaline is increased in victims of psychological trauma with PTSD. Well, it turns out that some drugs, heroin being the most effective, shut off the activity of the adrenaline center in the brain located in the brain stem, called the *locus coeruleus*. Other drugs that do this include benzodiazepines, such as Valium and alcohol. Our research studies showed that PTSD patients reported that these drugs help their symptoms (cocaine makes them worse). The problem is that sooner or later the consequences of drug usage catch up with them. In any case, this clear case of heroin helping PTSD symptoms led to what we called the "self-medication hypothesis of PTSD."

Substance abuse is not the only area where trauma victims have a disconnect. Trauma victims don't make the connection between the trauma in their lives and their behavior in many ways.

The first step in recovery is to educate your client about what effects psychological trauma has had upon them and their behavior. You probably know most of the mental health effects, but you might not know about some of the evidence showing that psychological trauma affects physical health in many ways. This will be covered in the next chapter.

CHAPTER 6: EFFECTS OF PSYCHOLOGICAL TRAUMA ON PHYSICAL HEALTH

Psychological trauma takes a toll on not only the mind and brain, but also the body. This can lead to a number of potentially disabling physical symptoms, like headaches, nausea, indigestion, and feelings of breathlessness, that don't always have a clear cause.

Psychological trauma can also be associated with potentially life-threatening disorders with clearly identifiable physical abnormalities, including cancer, heart disease, gastric ulcers and diabetes.

Finally, the functional pain disorders are defined as disorders with specific symptoms where an underlying medical cause is not easy to find. These disorders, which are very common, are often seen in people with a history of psychological trauma, although a trauma history is not necessary for their development. Functional pain disorders include irritable bowel syndrome (IBS), fibromyalgia, non-specific low back pain, chronic pelvic pain, and temporomandibular pain around the face and jaw, and are discussed in more detail later.

Psychological trauma can also be associated with somatization disorders, described in more detail below.

Stress and Heart Disease

Heart disease is the most common cause of death in the United States, and psychological trauma contributes to the development of heart disease in many people. The ancient Greeks, as well as many other cultures throughout history, believed the heart was the source of emotion. This idea has carried over into statements about someone dying of a broken heart, and similar expressions. The fact is this popular wisdom may not be so far from the truth.

Research done by us and others showed that emotional factors, including exposure to psychological trauma, play a role in heart disease. Repeated or chronic stress can have a wearing response on the heart, immune function, and metabolism of glucose, leading to chronic elevations in blood pressure and heart rate, problems with immune responses to infections, and elevations in blood sugar that may lead to diabetes. This is in part related to chronic elevations of the stress hormones, cortisol and adrenaline.

Psychological trauma makes you more reactive to minor stressors in life or reminders of your trauma, especially if you have PTSD or depression. These mental processes can trigger a rapid and reversible narrowing of the blood vessels of the heart, leading to what we call ischemia, which can cause chest pain or damage to the tissues of the heart.

Stress can also cause atherosclerosis, which is a build up in the walls of the blood vessels in the heart of fats (lipids), cholesterol, and white blood cells (the cells in the body that fight infections). With time, these atherosclerotic collections can harden, which is why they are called athero (which means pudding in Greek) sclerosis (which means hardened). These atherosclerotic plaques can become brittle and break, sometimes sending a piece of plaque downstream to lodge in the narrow part of the blood vessel, blocking blood flow to a part of the heart. When that happens, it causes the heart's muscle tissue to die, leading to a heart attack, which could be fatal.

How Does Psychological Trauma Cause Heart Disease?

How is it that psychological trauma can cause a physical disorder like heart disease?

There are a number of possible ways, including the chronic elevations in cortisol and adrenaline that can lead to chronically high blood pressure and heart rate, changes in blood sugar, or changes in the peripheral nervous system that controls the heart and blood vessels. Animal studies show that chronic stress actually damages the inside of the blood vessels of the heart, probably due to excessively high levels of adrenaline. Psychological trauma also affects immune function, which can affect the heart, leading to an increase in heart disease in people with PTSD and depression related to psychological trauma.

Based on our research, we think that psychological trauma leads to an over-reaction of the blood vessels, so that the muscles in the wall of the blood vessels become over-reactive. This can cause a stress-induced narrowing that decreases blood flow to certain parts of the heart, resulting in ischemia (which is a lessening of blood flow to a particular part of the body), and possibly heart attacks.

Increase in Heart Disease with Natural Disasters

When there is an emotionally stressful event, like natural or industrial disasters, or terrorist attacks, there is an increase in heart disease. This can be seen in an increase in admissions to the hospital for chest pain and heart attacks (see the chapter "Heart Disease and Depression" by Vaccarino and Bremner in Appendix D). Even things like major sporting events have been associated with an increase in admissions to the hospital for heart disease. For instance,

- In the week after the Northridge earthquake in the Los Angeles area in 1994, there was a 35% increase in people admitted to the hospital for heart attacks, and a five-fold increase in sudden cardiac deaths.

- After the World Trade Center terrorist attack in New York City on September 11, 2001, there was a 50% increase in heart disease in New York over the next three years.

Other studies show that people who've had a short-term increase in work load, such as a high pressure deadline, have a six-fold increase in the risk of having a heart attack during the next day.

Sudden stressors, even something like a surprise birthday party, can "stun" the heart, causing it to pump blood abnormally for a short period of time.

Studying the Effects of Stress on the Heart in the Laboratory

One thing we do in our research program at Emory University in Atlanta, GA, is see how people with heart disease react to stress. To do this, we bring them into the laboratory to do what we call a "mental stress test," using complicated and difficult things like having them do hard math problems, make speeches, or solve puzzles under time pressure. We then measure blood flow in the heart with a scanner.

Mental stress can cause a reduction in blood flow in the heart, or ischemia, in some people, in the same way that physical exercise can. At least one third of heart disease patients get ischemia during mental stress, usually without feeling any pain.

Even simple stresses of daily life can make the heart ischemic. In other words, a lot of people are walking around with potentially dangerous drops in blood flow to the heart when they get stressed out. This can happen multiple times per day, without their ever knowing about it. Our research studies showed that this is more common in people with psychological trauma in childhood and the diagnosis of PTSD or depression.

As well as ischemia, mental stress seems to affect the electrical properties of the heart. People with mental-stress-induced ischemia have an increase in heart attacks and risk of death related to a sudden stoppage of the heart due to problems with the electrical functioning of the heart. All kinds of stressors have been shown to affect heart function, including psychological trauma like childhood abuse, as well as stress at work and in the marriage, or the stress of having to care for a sick family member. These can all increase the risks of heart attacks and death from heart disease.

Functional Pain Disorders and Psychological Trauma

Psychological trauma is also associated with an increased risk for the development of functional pain disorders. These disorders are defined as ones that, after appropriate medical assessment, cannot be explained in terms of a conventionally defined medical disease based on specific biochemical or structural abnormalities.

Many times the functional pain disorders do not respond to conventional medical therapy. If your client does suffer from one, though, it is important for them to understand the symptoms so that they can get a handle on coping with them.

Although they are usually more common in people with psychological trauma, that doesn't necessarily mean they are always caused by psychological trauma, or that there aren't other contributing factors, like things in the environment, a history of physical injury, or genetic factors. Trauma may be one of many factors that contribute to the disorders, although not likely the only one (see "Combat-related Psychiatric Syndromes" in *Functional Pain Disorders* listed in Appendix D).

Irritable Bowel Syndrome

Irritable bowel syndrome (IBS) accounts for almost half of all visits to gastroenterologists, and is one of the most common gastrointestinal diseases.

IBS is characterized by abdominal pain and discomfort and associated alterations in bowel habits with no identifiable change in the function or structure of the bowels. Similar to other functional syndromes, IBS has been defined as "symptoms not explained by structural or biochemical abnormalities" and the diagnosis has been determined by symptom criteria (e.g., pain with bowel movements).

Patients with IBS more commonly report problems with sleep, sex drive, and a loss of energy, as well as headaches, back pain, muscle pain, pain while urinating, and a feeling of urinary urgency. IBS is felt to be related to a change in how the brain communicates with the bowels, which involves both processing of emotion and how the brain regulates the bowel through the peripheral nervous system.

One theory holds that IBS is related to stress, at least in some patients. Exposure to a threat is associated with changes in bowel function in animals, including

- an increase in defecation,

- changes in colonic motility,

- changes felt to be modulated by corticotropin releasing factor (CRF), and;

- autonomic nervous system influences on the gut.

Studies have shown an increase in childhood sexual abuse trauma and exposure to general traumatic events in IBS patients. Combat veterans, especially those with PTSD, have an increase in gastrointestinal symptoms and self-reported digestive diseases. Other studies have shown that parental style, specifically hostility and rejection from paternal figures, plays a greater role in the development of IBS than childhood sexual abuse. Rates of PTSD in IBS patients are typically higher than in the general population. An increase in symptoms of anxiety and depression, but not dissociation, has also been reported in IBS patients.

Fibromyalgia

Fibromyalgia, which affects about 5% of women and 2% percent of men, is associated with chronic widespread pain, diffuse tenderness, fatigue and sleep disturbance; diagnostic criteria require at least three months of widespread pain and pain upon digital palpation at no fewer than eleven of eighteen characteristic tender points.

Some studies have associated childhood physical abuse (but not childhood sexual abuse), or sexual assault in adulthood, with fibromyalgia. About half of fibromyalgia patients have PTSD. Fibromyalgia symptoms are also seen in at least a fifth of PTSD patients. Veterans deployed to the Gulf War had an increase in self-reported fibromyalgia (19% deployed versus 10% non-deployed).

PTSD patients with fibromyalgia symptoms have worse quality of life and more psychological distress than PTSD patients without fibromyalgia. Fibromyalgia patients also have increased rates of anxiety, depression and somatization.

Fibromyalgia is thought to be related at least in part to alterations in brain regions involved in pain and how they communicate with other parts of the body.

Low Back Pain

In the United States, back pain is the second most common symptom that drives people to go to the doctor. As with fibromyalgia and IBS, there is a lack of observable pathology to account for non-specific low back pain, treatment is difficult, and the relationship with emotional factors is not well defined.

Less than 15% of people with low back pain have an identifiable cause and treatment. This leaves a substantial proportion of people suffering back pain without any identifiable abnormality in their backs.

Prisoners of War (POWs) from Vietnam reported an increase in back problems compared to non-POW servicemen. Many returning Iraq veterans have both back pain and PTSD. They have high rates of pain related to mechanical wear and tear injuries from carrying more equipment than in prior wars (e.g., bullet proof vests) and jumping out of helicopters and armed vehicles. Low back pain and PTSD can maintain each other, with lack of mobility leading to increased avoidance, one of the symptoms of PTSD.

Chronic Pelvic Pain

Chronic pelvic pain is intermittent or continuous pain in the pelvic area that lasts at least three months.

Some people have thought of chronic pelvic pain as being a result of childhood sexual abuse. Although rates of childhood sexual trauma are higher in pelvic pain patients, exposure to childhood sexual trauma is not necessary for the development of the disorder. About half of patients with chronic pelvic pain also have PTSD. These patients also have an increase in other kinds of somatic problems.

Temporomandibular Joint Disorder (TMJD)

Temporomandibular joint disorder (TMJD) refers to pain in the jaw that can be caused by a number of factors, one of which is gnashing of teeth associated with stress. About 25% of patients with TMJD suffer from PTSD.

Somatoform Disorders

Somatoform disorders are described in the Diagnostic and Statistical Manual (DSM) of psychiatry as disorders where physical symptoms are not attributable to a known organic cause, and are not secondary to anxiety or depression. Somatization disorder involves at least eight physical symptoms in four bodily systems.

Somatization disorder patients have increased symptoms of dissociative amnesia, but not depersonalization, derealization or identify confusion or alteration. Somatization patients were found to have more history of emotional and physical abuse (but not sexual abuse) in childhood, plus more family conflict and less family cohesion.

Psychosomatic Disorders

Another term we use for all of these disorders (including the somatoform disorders and the functional pain disorders) is "psychosomatic disorders." The medical field, however, has evolved from the "it's all in your head" way of thinking to realizing that these disorders often involve a complex interchange between emotion, brain function, and function of peripheral organs, like the heart and the stomach. Multiple factors, including childhood environment, psychological trauma, physical injuries, and genetics likely play a role in these disorders.

The Complex Interplay of Stress, Mind, Brain and Body

The functional pain disorders often occur with each other and with stress-related psychiatric disorders like PTSD and depression, as well as chronic fatigue syndrome and headache. This may represent a common etiology (e.g., stress, common genetic factors, common changes in the brain), or the fact that they are involved in each other's etiology (e.g., pain leads to depression, or depression is involved in maintenance of pain after minor injury).

Sometimes symptoms of dissociation, which were reviewed in the previous chapter, are associated with functional pain syndromes. Symptoms of dissociation can resemble symptoms of a disorder called conversion disorder, which, like depersonalization, can involve distortions of how people perceive their own bodies. In conversion disorder, people may develop symptoms of losing sensation or function of an arm or leg, even though there is no identifiable medical cause. This is called "glove and stocking anesthesia," because there may be a pattern of loss of sensation that is like a glove, while the nerves are not distributed that way in the body.

Since PTSD and depression often occur with the functional pain disorders, it is likely there is some link with psychological trauma, at least in some people. However, the fact that not all patients with functional pain disorders have a history of psychological trauma, nor for that matter the diagnosis of PTSD or depression, suggests that psychological trauma is not essential for the development of chronic pain disorders.

Functional pain disorders are often associated with psychiatric symptoms from the attendant psychological trauma. We cover this in more detail in the next chapter.

CHAPTER 7: EFFECTS OF PSYCHOLOGICAL TRAUMA ON THE INDIVIDUAL

The U.S. spends $2,100 a year on research on HIV/AIDS for every person suffering from these disorders in this country, and only $18 per person with depression. This is in spite of the fact that depression is much more common than HIV/AIDS. That means that if your clients are suffering from depression or PTSD related to psychological trauma, they've got an uphill battle. This chapter gives some tips on how to help their clients in their recovery.

Educate Your Clients About Psychological Trauma

Knowledge is power, and the more your clients know about the behavioral effects of psychological trauma the better off they'll be. Know thyself. That was the motto of the great Greek philosopher, Socrates, who lived over 2,000 years ago, but whose words are as relevant now as they were back then.

I think it's a good idea to educate your clients about the symptoms of PTSD, depression, and dissociation

Why do I think that education is so important?

Because by learning about the symptoms that can be caused by psychological trauma, including both the mental and the physical consequences, your client can recognize the source. They stop attributing things to the fact that they are evil, have a bad character, or have done something wrong, and can recognize that their behavior is related to their life experiences. It also helps to educate their family members.

Negative Soundtracks

Many clients with a history of psychological trauma, especially emotional abuse, have a negative soundtrack running in their minds that comments on themselves and their behavior. It might be something like "you're no good," "get over it" or "you don't appreciate what you have." I write down the content of the negative soundtrack with my clients. Sometimes it is very difficult for them and I will keep the copy on their behalf and when they are ready we will take it out and read it. Usually the language is a copy of the kinds of things the abusive parent said.

Another nifty trick is to tell your client to say the comments in their mind with a cartoon voice, like Mickey Mouse or Donald Duck.

Childhood sexual abuse survivors may think there was something wrong with them that led to their being singled out for abuse, and their abusers may have reinforced these ideas by calling them stupid, or a slut, or a mistake, or some other negative thing.

Similarly, rape survivors may feel it was their fault for having crossed that parking lot alone, or having too many beers, or going out with that guy when they should have known better, or wearing that suggestive dress, etc.. Society and the legal system reinforce these attitudes by immediately asking questions about the sexual practices of the victimized woman. Muslim countries ostracize rape victims, which causes them to deny that rape ever happened.

It helps to correct your client's inaccurate and unhelpful cognitions. If they were raped in a parking lot, why is it their fault for walking alone at night? Rape is illegal, so the only person who was at fault was the rapist.

Other types of negative cognitions have to do with cause and effect. If your client was in a car accident and was severely injured, that doesn't mean that every time they drive a car they will get into another accident. If they were attacked in a dark alley, that doesn't mean that every time they go into a dark place they will be attacked. You can help them understand that their anxiety and fears are not reality based, and help them to overcome those fears.

Anniversary Reactions

Traumatized people often have what we call anniversary reactions linked to the time when a traumatic event happened to them; the date when their trauma occurred comes around, and they may start to feel worse.

The most famous anniversary in the United States is September 11, 2001, when terrorists flew airplanes into the World Trade Center in New York City, killing several thousand people. Thousands of people in America feel much worse around this time of year. This is one type of anniversary reaction, but anniversary reactions can come in many forms.

Many Vietnam combat veterans have an anniversary reaction around the time of year of the Tet offensive, which occurred on January 30, 1968. This was the date on which the North Vietnamese launched a massive offensive against the South Vietnamese and American forces, and has become a negative anniversary for many veterans of the Vietnam War.

Parents who lose their children have anniversary reactions for the time of their death, or maybe even their birthdays. People tend to become more symptomatic in the weeks leading up to the anniversary, and peak at the time of the anniversary. Many people don't even recognize what's happening.

How do you help your clients deal with anniversary reactions?

- First of all, help them recognize that they exist.

- Then encourage them to prepare themselves in advance to deal with them effectively.

- They should not try and ignore it because it will come up and hit them in the face.

- If they need to they can tell people in their life that this time of year is difficult, and they need to be alone more, or that they may be more difficult to live with, or need more attention and support than usual.

Break the Cycle of Abuse

We know that abuse victims are more likely to go on to abuse their own children. The reasons for this are complex but probably include the fact that

- parents have learned parenting (good and bad) from their own parents,

- victims feel a sense of powerlessness that they may compensate for (inappropriately) by manipulating powerless children when they grow up,

- an inability to cope with the stressful behavior of their children causes them to lash out, or

- the increase in drug use associated with their victimization impairs their judgment and removes inhibitions of behavior.

Some abuse victims recognize this and do not want to take the chance of having their own children, but they don't need to go that far. They just need to learn to recognize that they may have trouble coping, that there may be times they need to get help in order to cope with the stress of parenting. Learn to take a walk or count to ten .

Effects of Trauma on Psychological Development in Childhood

One of the things I consider when evaluating trauma patients is the phase of development when the person first experience psychological trauma, and whether it continued into later phases of development.

This is important because early childhood is a significant time for the development of identity, and trauma can have a profound effect on the psychological development of children.

Stressful events or disruptions in the maternal–infant bond can lead to problems with the development of a stable and secure self-identity. For these reasons, trauma that occurs early in life leads to more problems with identity as the child matures. This can contribute to identity confusion in adulthood, and, at its most extreme, personality disorders and dissociative identity disorder.

Patients with early trauma also develop multifactorial psychiatric disorders, which can include depression, somatic disorders, and alcohol and substance abuse, the trauma spectrum disorders outlined in *Does Stress Damage the Brain?* It is important to identify all of the disorders from which a trauma patient is suffering and to identify treatments for all aspects of those disorders.

Patients without a history of childhood trauma who are traumatized in adulthood — whether from a car accident, natural disaster, or events akin to those of September 11 — look similar, regardless of the trauma type. These patients typically have a more "pure" presentation of PTSD symptoms, with increased arousal and vigilance, but fewer of the depression and personality symptoms that early trauma patients develop.

These adult trauma patients respond well to cognitive behavioral therapies that concentrate on processing of the actual traumatic event, with a desensitization to aspects of the event that increase arousal and intrusive memories. With time, the traumatic event is processed both emotionally and cognitively, and negative cognitions and other unhelpful cognitive processes are corrected — the event is placed in a proper context and integrated into the patient's catalogue of life experiences.

These patients can also benefit from medication treatment in conjunction with behavioral treatments, such as SSRIs (Selective Serotonin Reuptake Inhibitors).

Early trauma patients, on the other hand, have a more complicated presentation and do not always benefit from traditional cognitive behavioral therapies. For these patients, the reintroduction of traumatic memories may be associated with an increase in dissociation, negative emotions, or identity confusions and crises that the patient cannot control. In such situations, retrieving traumatic memories for attempted therapeutic benefit is not always helpful.

Some early trauma patients need long-term therapies aimed at psychological support, supplemented with medications where appropriate. Many early trauma patients who have disabling psychiatric symptoms are treated with multiple medications, which may include SSRI and a mood-stabilizing agent like valproic acid (Valproate) or carbamazepine (Tegretol).

Although patients who have their first traumatic event in adulthood look very similar in terms of their symptoms, regardless of trauma type, there are some aspects of trauma that influence what kinds of symptoms they might have. This is largely related to different trauma types leading to different types of fear reactions. For example, women who are victims of sexual assault will be more likely to have problems with sexual intimacy, related to fear responses associated to sexual activity. Conversely, motor vehicle accident victims may have fear responses related to approaching an automobile.

The Meaning of Psychological Trauma

The response to trauma is also influenced by factors such as the meaning the event had for the individual, and social and cultural factors related to the event.

Children who are sexually abused by a biological parent whom they trust and rely on for caregiving and support will have a different response than someone who is victimized by a stranger. Also, patients who are not able to talk about their trauma in a supportive environment and social context may have additional suffering.

Many veterans of the Vietnam War, upon returning to the United States, did not find their country to be supportive of the sacrifices they made. Similarly, in Muslim countries there is great shame for women to admit they have been victims of sexual assault. Therefore, in countries such as Bosnia where there was systematic rape of the female population, many families do not want to talk about their traumatic experiences.

The Neuroscience of Early Interventions for Trauma

Appropriate treatment of trauma victims may require rapid interventions soon after the trauma.

We know from animal studies that memories are not immediately engraved in the mind — it can take a month or more before they become indelible. For instance, animals that undergo lesions of the hippocampus within the first month after an aversive memory lose all recall of what happened.

During this time period, the memories continue to be susceptible to modification; this time period is known as memory consolidation. However, if you wait too long, a month or more, it is no longer possible to erase the negative memory simply by lesioning the hippocampus. At that point, the memory becomes engraved in the long-term memory storage areas in the cerebral cortex, the outermost part of the brain.

After the memory has become engraved in long-term memory storage, it is indelible and no longer easily amenable to modification. This may represent the case of, for example, combat veterans with longstanding PTSD, for whom no amount of treatment is able to erase the traumatic memories of their combat experiences.

That is why it is important to intervene early, before the traumatic memories become indelible.

Animal studies indicate that early interventions will be beneficial before traumatic memories become firmly engraved in the mind. We know from these studies that medications given before exposure to trauma — including valium-type medications, antidepressants, opiates, and alcohol — can diminish or prevent the long-term behavioral effects of stressors.

Clinical studies also show that some medications given before a trauma can prevent long-term psychopathology. For example, in a study of people exposed to a hotel fire, those individuals who were intoxicated with alcohol at the time of the fire had a better psychiatric outcome than did those who were not. This may mean that it is better to get treatment before they are even diagnosed with having a psychiatric disorder, which often requires having symptoms for at least a month.

Trauma and Grief

Sometimes after psychological trauma there is a blockage of the normal grief reaction. Psychiatrists are increasingly talking about grief as evidence of a mental condition, but in fact it is a normal part of the healing process after we lose someone close to us.

Elisabeth Kubler-Ross wrote a book in 1969 called *On Death and Dying* that remains to this day a classic guidebook on the grief process. She described five stages of grief that follow the sudden loss of a loved one, like a spouse, parent, close friend, or child:

- The first stage is denial. You are in a state of shock. You say there must have been a mistake, or maybe I heard it wrong. Maybe someone is playing a joke. I just saw that person yesterday, and they looked fine.

- With time the reality sets in that the person really is gone, and then denial turns to anger. Why couldn't the doctors have done something to save their life? Why didn't someone call 911 right away? Why did the person have to do x or y, thus putting themselves at risk? Why is God so unjust?

- The next stage is bargaining, where you may try to talk to God and make a deal to bring the person back, or maybe you make a promise to change your life or do some charitable activity in exchange for the loved one coming back.

- When it becomes clear that bargaining is useless, the person who was left behind succumbs to depression.

- But finally, maybe weeks or months later, arrives acceptance of the loss, and the realization that this is just

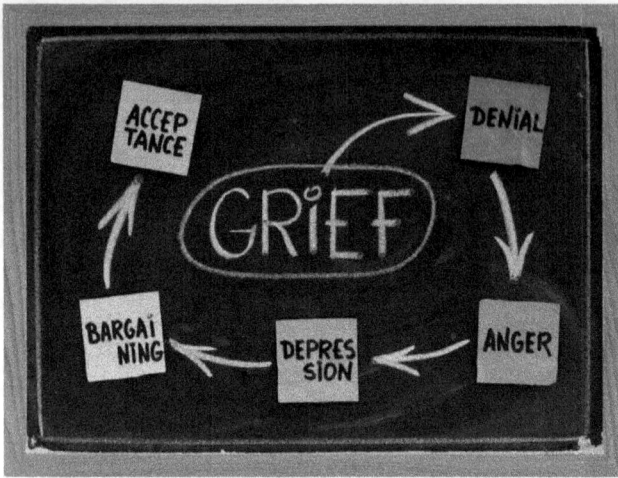

FIGURE 11: STAGES OF GRIEF

part of life, no matter how unfair it seems.

Another theory for grief that many people have found helpful is J. William Worden's book, *Grief Counseling and Grief Therapy: A Handbook for the Mental Health Practitioner.* Worden's approach is proactive.

Worden recommends four tasks to complete the process of mourning. He thinks that the path to recovery is more of a circle than a straight line. He says that you can't put your grief work on a schedule. Everyone's different and there are so many things involved that you may think you are done but then you get surprised by how it seems like your grief is circling back again and starting all over. This is the way the grief process works.

The First Task: The first task Worden identifies is "To accept the reality of the loss" which includes not just the fact of the loss but also the significance of the loss. Simple things like going to a funeral or talking (and thinking) about the person in the past tense help us accept the reality of the loss. Even though you talk about someone in the past tense, however, it may not hit right away how significant the loss really is. For instance, people might downplay how important that person was to them, which is a way of denying the impact the loss has had or will have on them.

Often a big hurdle to overcome in the grieving process is coming to terms with how the person died. If someone kills themselves it is common for people to feel like that person didn't want to be with them anymore. Not only do you have to mourn the loss of your loved one, you also have to come to terms with what the suicide means to you personally. Death by drug or alcohol overdose is similar in that it is a self-inflicted death, and may have a stigma that makes it hard to be open and talk about your feelings. Maybe your loved one died in a foreign combat zone, or maybe they disappeared and their body was never found. What happens to the body is very important. The ancient Greeks fought whole battles over trying to get the bodies of their dead soldiers back from their enemies!

The Second Task: The second task is "To work through the pain of grief". Each person will experience a range of different emotions after someone dies. None of these feelings are abnormal or wrong, although some may be more difficult to resolve. Sadness, fear, loneliness, despair, hopelessness, anger, guilt, blame, shame and even relief are all emotions you might have to contend with. As we will be going over later the "T" in START Now is for Talking about your feelings, which makes you realize that they are real. Here in the USA we don't do a very good job of dealing with death, and a lot of people don't feel comfortable talking about it or feel like they might say the wrong thing. They might think that if they just ignore the fact that someone died the uncomfortableness will just go away. It is never a good idea, though, to deny or avoid our feelings about the death of a loved one. A simple but good thing to say is "I'm sorry for your loss." Or maybe you can add "I'll be thinking about you." That is not patronizing but it expresses that you care and acknowledges to the person the importance of what happened. Reach out and find the positive support you need to talk about your feelings (as you will learn later, "S" is for Seek Safety and Support). You can also take Action or practice Altruism (the "A" in, guess what?) like setting up a scholarship or memorial in honor of the person you lost..

The Third Task: Task three is "To adjust to an environment in which the deceased is missing". It can take a long time to get used to the person not being around, not only with your feelings, but things like not having another person in the house, or having to learn how to do the finances if that person always took care of that..

The Fourth Task: Finally, task four is "To find an enduring connection with the deceased while embarking on a new life". Worden recognized that people need to continue to feel connected with the person who died. He would never say, "Just snap out of it". You can tell how far along you are on this task by observing how difficult or easy it is to have thoughts and memories of the person who died.

When someone dies you might feel like your life has stopped or that you will never be able to feel joy or pleasure again. Don't worry, this is a normal reaction, and it may take a long time to go away. Again, don't put a time schedule on it. However, if you follow the points in this book, you will one day again be able to enjoy things. Trust us!

It is important that you allow yourself to express your feelings, including sorrow and sadness. If you don't, you will never regain the emotional equilibrium that allows you to feel extreme joy. Numbing out the grief has a way of taking out all feelings with it. Remember, only you can feel your feelings. Don't let other people tell you how you feel. And most importantly of all, don't listen to people who tell you to "just get over it."

Many times victims of psychological trauma get stuck in the grieving process. They are so overwhelmed by the tragedy that they can't move through the normal grieving process. Or maybe they are in dangerous circumstances, like a war zone, and don't have the opportunity to grieve. Children who are in an abusive family are not encouraged to express their feelings.

Many of the combat veterans with PTSD I have treated over the years describe a feeling of numbness when someone in their family dies. As one vet told me, "they have to get in line to be grieved for, because I have a whole string of people I never grieved for who died in Vietnam."

The reality is that it might take up to a year to recover from devastating loss, as described in the book *Healing After Loss, Daily Meditations for Recovery from Grief*, by Martha Whitmore Hickman. That book has a meditation on grief and loss, sometimes with quotes from literature, for every day of the week. I recommend that book for your clients who experience a loss. The can read each day's entry for every day of the week.

Grieving clients need to express their feelings, including sorrow and sadness. If they don't, they will never regain the emotional equilibrium that allows them to feel extreme joy. Because numbing out the grief has a way of taking out all feelings with it.

Many times victims of psychological trauma get stuck in the grieving process. They are so overwhelmed by the tragedy that they can't move through the normal grieving process. Or maybe they are in dangerous circumstances, like a war zone, and don't have the opportunity to grieve. Children who are in an abusive family are not encouraged to express their feelings.

Many of the combat veterans with PTSD I have treated over the years describe a feeling of numbness when someone in their family dies. As one vet told me, "they have to get in line to be grieved for, because I have a whole string of people I never grieved for who died in Vietnam."

CHAPTER 8: MEDICATIONS FOR TRAUMA-RELATED MENTAL CONDITIONS

Prescription medications can be an important part of the recovery process for individuals with stress-related mental disorders. Medications commonly used for these disorders include the antidepressants, antipsychotics, benzodiazepines, insomnia medications, anti-anxiety medications and mood stabilizers. Within the antidepressants there are the original drugs, called tricyclics, the second generation of selective serotonin inhibitors (SSRIs), and the third generation of serotonin/norepinephrine reuptake inhibitors (SNRIs). Antipsychotic medications include the first generation and second generation or "atypicals." An older class of medication not used as much any more are the monoamine reuptake inhibitors (MAOIs). Insomnia medications include benzodiazepines and the so-called "z" drugs. Medications for anxiety include serotonin 1A receptor agonists like buspirone and benzodiazepines. Medications developed for the treatment of epilepsy like lamotrigine and valproic acid are also used as mood stabilizers for trauma patients.

Antidepressants

Although the antidepressants were originally developed for the treatment of depression, as their name implies, they have since been found to be useful in the treatment of other disorders related to stress, and PTSD. In fact, as I outline in my book *Does Stress Damage the Brain* (2002) there is considerable Truth is, there is a lot of overlap in the symptoms of mental conditions related to stress, and it is not uncommon for drugs developed for one problem to work for another.

Tricyclic Antidepressant Medications

The first antidepressant drugs were called the tricyclics, because their chemical structure included three rings. The tricyclics work mainly on the adrenaline, or norepinephrine, system of the brain.

The tricyclic antidepressants include imipramine and amitriptyline. They are not used as commonly as they used to be because of side effects related to the cholinergic nervous system, including:

- dry mouth,

- problems urinating,

- blurred vision,

- decreased bowel function, and;

- possibly effects on heart function.

These side effects are not long lasting and are usually only seen in the first weeks of treatment. However, when newer antidepressants came on the market, they largely replaced the tricyclics, although some patients may specifically have a good response to them. Claims that the newer SSRIs are more efficacious are not in fact borne out by the research. Tricyclics and SSRIs work equally well.

Antidepressant Medications With Other Mechanisms of Action

Some antidepressant medications act on other brain chemical systems besides norepinephrine and serotonin, such as dopamine. Dopamine transmission is associated with increased energy and feelings of euphoria. Medications that stimulate dopamine such as bupropion (Wellbutrin) (Wellbutrin) increase the levels of dopamine in the brain. Marketed under the name Zyban bupropion is also used as a smoking cessation drug. Side effects include:

- weight loss

- restlessness

- rarely, at high doses, seizures

Other antidepressant medications that also work on dopamine and/or do not have specific actions on norepinephrine or serotonin include:

- trazodone (Desyrel)

- maprotiline (Ludiomil)

- mirtazapine (Remeron)

These antidepressants also don't have as many anticholinergic side effects and effects on the heart and blood pressure as the tricyclics. They also don't have as many sexual side effects as the SSRIs (see below). Trazodone can rarely cause priapism (extended painful erection that requires emergency treatment). It is often used to treat insomnia in patients with PTSD and depression. Side effects of mirtazapine include:

- sweating

- tiredness

- strange dreams

- elevation of lipids

- weight gain

- upset stomach

- anxiety

- agitation

Selective Serotonin Reuptake Inhibitors (SSRIs)

The selective serotonin reuptake inhibitors (SSRIs) block the protein on the neuron that takes serotonin   back up into the neuron from the synapse, or space between the neurons. Thus they effectively increase serotonin levels in the brain.

SSRIs include:

- paroxetine (Paxil)

- fluoxetine (Prozac)

- sertraline (Zoloft)

- fluvoxamine (Luvox)

- citalopram (Celexa)

- escitalopram (Lexapro)

Paroxetine and sertraline are approved for the treatment of PTSD by the FDA. All of them are approved for the treatment of depression. An important possible side effect of the SSRIs is loss of libido or other sexual side effects. Patients should be encouraged to tell their doctors about this. The SSRIs have fewer anti-cholinergic side effects than the tricyclics. Side effects can include:

- nausea,

- diarrhea,

- headache,

- insomnia, and;

- agitation

If patients suddenly stop taking SSRIs or increase the dose too rapidly it can result in suicidal thoughts.

Dual Reuptake Inhibitors (SNRIs)

The serotonin and norepinephrine reuptake inhibitors (SNRIs) include venlafaxine (Effexor) and duloxetine (Cymbalta). They work to boost both the serotonin and norepinephrine neurotransmitter systems.

In general, venlafaxine and duloxetine seem to work better for depression than SSRIs and tricyclics, but they also increase the risk for suicidal thoughts compared to the SSRIs and tricyclics, although these occur rarely.

When a number of studies were looked at together, overall, venlafaxine had a success rate of 74% — that's statistically significantly better than SSRIs, with a 61% success rate, and tricyclics, with a 58% success rate. Although tricyclics work just as well for depression as the SSRIs patients are more likely to stop taking them because of side effects than the SSRIs. Possible side effects include:

- dizziness, constipation, dry mouth, headache, changes in sleep, or

- more rarely a serotonin syndrome, with restlessness, shivering and sweating.

- A decrease in saliva can cause cavities.

• Venlafaxine has been associated with a dose dependent increase in blood pressure.

• Venlafaxine seems to carry the greatest risk of suicidality amongst all of the antidepressants, with three-fold increased risk of attempted or completed suicides.

Antidepressant and Mood Stabilizer Medications: Use and Risks

Drug	Use	Common, benign side effects	Serious side effects	Life threatening side effects	Reasons not to take
TRICYCLICS Moderate Risk					
doxepin (Sinequaan) or imipramine (Tofranil)	Major depression	Dry mouth, constipation, memory, blurred vision, urination, sexual function	Blood pressure changes,	Heart arrhythmias, overdose	Heart condition
amitriptyline (Elavil) or amoxapine (Asendin)	Major depression	Dry mouth, constipation, memory, blurred vision, urination, sexual function	Blood pressure changes,	Heart arrhythmias, overdose	Heart condition, seizures, glaucoma

Drug	Use	Common, benign side effects	Serious side effects	Life threatening side effects	Reasons not to take
Norepinephrine Reuptake Inhibitors *Low Risk*					
desipramine (Norpramin) *or* nortriptyline (Aventyl, Pamelor) *or* amoxapine (Ascendin)	Major depression	Dry mouth, constipation, memory	blurred vision, urination, sexual function	Heart arrhythmias, seizures	Heart condition, seizures, glaucoma
clomipramine (Anafranil)	OCD	Dry mouth, constipation, memory	blurred vision, urination, sexual function	Heart arrhythmias, seizures	Heart condition, seizures, glaucoma
MAO Inhibitors *Moderate Risk*					
phenalzine (Nardil) *or* tranylcypromine (Parnate)	Major depression	constipation, blurred vision, urination, sexual function	Dizziness, headache, insomnia	Wine and cheese hypertensive crisis, liver damage, anemia	Liver disease, heart failure, pheochromocytoma, children
Quatrocyclics *Low Risk*					
mirtazapine (Remeron)	Major depression	Shivering, fatigue, nightmares, weight gain, anxiety, dry mouth, constipati	Lipid elevations, swelling, muscle pain	Trouble breathing, sore throat	Kidney or liver disease, MAOI

Drug	Use	Common, benign side effects	Serious side effects	Life threatening side effects	Reasons not to take
		on			
maprotiline (Ludiomil)	Major depression	Dry mouth, drowsiness, nausea, vomiting	Rash, swelling	Seizures, hallucinations, irregular heart rate, jaundice	Liver disease, MAOI
Selective Serotonin Reuptake Inhibitors (SSRI) *Low Risk*					
paroxetine (Paxil)	Major depression, panic, OCD, PTSD, GAD	Nausea, diarrhea, headache, insomnia	Decreased libido, akathisia	Suicidal thoughts, mood swings with dose change	Allergic reaction, MAOI
sertraline (Zoloft)	Major depression, panic, OCD, PTSD, GAD	Nausea, diarrhea, headache, insomnia	Decreased libido, akathisia	suicidal thoughts, mood swings with dose change, bleeding	Allergic reaction, MAOI
fluoxetine (Prozac)	Major depression and OCD	Nausea, diarrhea, headache, insomnia	Decreased libido, akathisia	Suicidal thoughts, mood swings with dose change	Allergic reaction, MAOI
fluvoxamine (Luvox)	Major depression	Nausea, diarrhea, headache, insomnia	Decreased libido, akathisia	Suicidal thoughts, mood swings with dose change	Allergic reaction, MAOI
Other Antidepressan					

Drug	Use	Common, benign side effects	Serious side effects	Life threatening side effects	Reasons not to take
ts					
bupropion (Wellbutrin, Zyban)	Depression, smoking cessation	Weight loss, restlessness, dry mouth, insomnia, con-stipation, nausea, vomiting		Seizures	Seizure disorder, allergic to medication
trazodone (Desyrel)	Major depression	Dizziness, constipation, dry mouth, headache	Priapism	Allergic reaction, irregular heart rate	Allergy to medication, pregnancy, acute heart disease
Dual Uptake Inhibitors					
venlafaxine (Effexor)	Major depression	Restlessness, shivering, constipation, nausea, headache	Sexual dysfunction, hypertension, muscle cramp	Suicidality, stomach bleeding, allergic reaction	Allergy to drug, MAOI
duloxetine (Cymbalta)	Major depression	Constipation, nausea, diarrhea, vomiting, dry mouth	Sexual dysfunction, blurred vision, muscle pain, dizziness	Stomach bleeding, liver damage	Allergy to drug, MAOI
Mood stabilizers					
lithium (Lithobid)	Bipolar disorder	Nausea, tremor, weight gain, diarrhea,	Blurred vision, stomach upset	Change in renal function	Heart disease, renal disease, brain damage, diuretics

Drug	Use	Common, benign side effects	Serious side effects	Life threatening side effects	Reasons not to take
		thirst			
valproic acid (Valproate, Depakene, Depakote)	Bipolar disorder	Mood change, anorexia, nausea, trembling	Rash, dizziness	Liver failure, birth defects, bleeding, pancreatitis	Liver disease, pregnancy, breast feeding
carbamazepine (Tegretol)	Bipolar disorder	Dizziness, drowsiness, nausea, vomiting	Confusion, depression, hallucina-tions	Bone marrow suppression, heart failure, liver dysfunction	Hypersensitivity, pregnancy, breast feeding, Allergy to medication
topiramate (Topomax)	Bipolar disorder	Dizziness, nervousness, headache, irritability	Confusion, aggression	Low blood sugar, blurred vision	Allergy to medication
lamotrigine (Lamictal)	Bipolar disorder	Dizziness, headache, sleepiness, nausea, vomiting	Blurred vision,	Steven Johnson syndrome	Allergy to medication
gabapentin (Neurontin)	Bipolar disorder	Dizziness, headache, sleepiness, nausea, vomiting	Blurred vision	Eye movements	Allergy to medication

FIGURE 12: ANTIDEPRESSANTS AND MOOD STABILIZERS: USES AND MAJOR RISKS

All medication tables are adapted from BEFORE YOU TAKE THAT PILL, by J. Douglas Bremner, © 2008 J. Douglas Bremner, used by permission of Avery Publishing, an imprint of the Penguin Group (see Appendix D).

Animal studies have shown that antidepressants have effects on parts of the brain involved in the stress response. SSRIs increase branching and growth of brain cells, or neurons, in the hippocampus. Treatment with the SSRI paroxetine (Paxil) in PTSD patients for a year resulted in a 5% increase in hippocampal volume measured with magnetic resonance imaging (MRI) and a 35% improvement in hippocampal-based memory function (for example, the ability to remember a paragraph or a list of words) as measured with neuropsychological testing. These patients felt that treatment with paroxetine led to a significant improvement in their ability to work and function in their lives. They were able to concentrate and remember things much better than before treatment with medication.

The Story of Jeff, with PTSD

One of the patients who was treated with paroxetine in one of our studies was a man named Jeff. Here's his story:

Jeff had been a cop in the Bridgeport, Connecticut, police force for twenty years. When he entered our study, he had reached a crisis point where he couldn't cope with his daily memories of a traumatic event that happened fifteen years before. His wife told him he should get counseling right away.

The morning of the incident, he took a call at concerning a suicide attempt. It was only four blocks away.

When he entered the house, a woman was screaming, "My son hurt himself, he didn't mean it, you've got to help him."

The father was very silent.

A five-year-old girl was crying and saying, "Help my brother, he's hurt."

Jeff entered the room. What had been a seventeen-year-old boy was lying on his bed with a shotgun on his chest. His face looked normal, but the top of his head was a cavity. He had literally blown his brains out. The boy's body was making a gasping sound as if he were breathing. As Jeff stood there, some of the brains sticking to the ceiling fell on his shoulder.

Following this incident, Jeff was bothered daily by memories of the event. He said, "I drift from one thing to another. Nothing seems to have any meaning anymore. I feel as if my life will end tomorrow, but I don't care."

Jeff would think over and over about how this thing happened, how it could have been prevented. The boy was depressed because he had acne, and thought a girl he liked wouldn't like him in turn. Jeff would ponder about how this could be his own son. He was tormented by his thoughts.

Sometimes, when he was reliving the event, he wasn't aware of anything around him. He tried to talk about it, he tried to be a tough cop and hold it in, but nothing relieved his anguish.

We started Jeff on Paxil at a variable dose. Within six weeks, Jeff showed an improvement in a number of PTSD symptoms, including intrusive symptoms like recurrent mental images of his trauma. He appeared to have an almost complete resolution of the symptoms that were causing him so much distress.

Other Medications for Treatment of Psychological Trauma

Other medications outside of the antidepressant class have been found to be useful for PTSD and depression:

• The anti-hypertension drug, prazosin (Minipres), has been shown in research studies to improve both symptoms of PTSD as well as nightmares and insomnia.

• We have had good results with the epilepsy drug, phenytoin (Dilantin), which has also been shown to block the effects of stress on the brain in animal studies, and which we have shown to increase brain volumes in PTSD patients.

• Some studies have shown that the beta blocker drug, propranolol, used to treat hypertension, can prevent the development of chronic PTSD when given soon after the trauma.

While medication may be a good start in itself, it's usually not enough. The best approach is usually to combine medication treatment with psychotherapy.

You can read more about medication treatment of PTSD and depression in *Before You Take That Pill: Why the Drug Industry May Be Bad For Your Health*, published by Penguin in 2008.

Antipsychotic Medication

Although designed for the treatment of schizophrenia, many doctors use antipsychotic medications for the treatment of stress-related psychiatric disorders. Studies have shown that the antipsychotics (also known as neuroleptics) can be useful as add on treatments to antidepressants for treatment resistant PTSD and depression, although they have some worrisome side effects including weight gain, diabetes, and tardive dyskinesia (a twitching in the face or other areas). Some studies show that the addition of antipsychotics leads to a small but statistically significant improvement in depression, although for every person who gets better, one develops the disturbing symptom of akathisia (a feeling like you want to jump

102

out of your skin). Fortunately, this symptom goes away when the drug is stopped the drug.

You may have seen advertisements on television for antipsychotic drugs like Abilify (aripiprazole) used in the treatment of depression. They show happy people floating out to their mailboxes, followed by an announcer reading a huge list of possible side effects as fast as he can (and the volume decreases dramatically.)

The original group of antipsychotic medications are now called the typical antipsychotics, the first in that class being chlorpromazine (Thorazine). Its discovery half a century ago allowed many people institutionalized for years for schizophrenia to move outside of the hospital.

The typical antipsychotic medications block the dopamine 2 receptor in the brain, which is involved in the symptoms of psychosis. Other first generation antipsychotics include thioridazine (Mellaril), perphenazine (Trilafon), fluphenazine (Prolixin), haloperidol (Haldol), loxapine (Loxatane), and thiothixene (Navane).

The typical antipsychotics can be associated with troubling side effects that are worse than with the antidepressants:

- extra-pyramidal side effects (involuntary muscle movements), including Parkinsonism, with tremor, rigidity, and shuffling gait;

- akathisia, a feeling of internal stiffness or restlessness that can be very uncomfortable, or dyskinesia, a painful stiffening of the muscles.

- Tardive Dyskinesia, which involves twitching, jerking movements, and lip smacking, of the lips, mouth, and arms.

- anti-cholinergic side effects including confusion, memory problems, dry mouth, sedation, and a lowering of the blood pressure.

The newer generation of antipsychotics are called the atypical antipsychotics. In addition to dopamine they block other receptors like the serotonin 2A receptors. This possibly explains why they are not as commonly associated with extra pyramidal side effects.

Atypical antipsychotic drugs include olanzapine (Zyprexa), risperidone (Risperdal), ziprasidone (Geodon), quetiapine (Seroquel), and aripiprazole (Abilify). These medications have not, however, been clearly been shown to work better than the typical antipsychotics. Side effects of atypical antipsychotics include

- drowsiness,

- drops in blood pressure,

- weight gain, and

- decreased sweating which may increase the risk of heat stroke.

The most worrisome possible side effects of the newer atypical antipsychotics is an impairment in glucose (sugar) metabolism, which increases the risk of weight gain and Type II diabetes.

Antipsychotic Medications: Uses and Risks

Drug	Indication	Common, benign side effects	Serious side effects	Life threatening side effects	Reasons not to take
Typical Antipsychotics *Medium Risk*					

Drug	Indication	Common, benign side effects	Serious side effects	Life threatening side effects	Reasons not to take
chlorpromazine (Thorazine) *or* fluphenazine (Prolixin) *or* haloperidol (Haldol) *or* loxapine (Loxatane) *or* thioridazine (Mellaril) *or* thiothixene (Navane)	Schizophrenia	Confusion, dry mouth, memory problems, sedation	Parkinsonism, tremor, rigidity, akathisia, dyskinesia, tardive dyskinesia	Orthostatic hypotension, neuroleptic malignant syndrome	Hypersensitivity
mesoridazine (Serentil) *or* perphenazine (Trilafon)	Schizophrenia	Confusion, dry mouth, memory problems, sedation	Parkinsonism, tremor, rigidity, akathisia, dyskinesia, tardive dyskinesia	Orthostatic hypotension, neuroleptic malignant syndrome Prolongation of QT interval with cardiac death	Prolonged QT interval or heart disease; hypersensitivity
Atypical Antipsychotics *Medium Risk*					
olanzepine (Zyprexa) *or* risperidone (Risperdal)	Schizophrenia	Drowsiness, decreased sweating, headache, nausea, vomiting	Weight gain, constipation	Neuroleptic malignant syndrome, diabetes	Hypersensitivity
ziprasidone (Geodon)	Schizophrenia	Drowsiness,	Weight gain,	Neuroleptic malignant	Hypersensitivity

Drug	Indication	Common, benign side effects	Serious side effects	Life threatening side effects	Reasons not to take
		decreased sweating, headache, nausea, vomiting	constipation	syndrome Increases QT interval with risk of cardiac death	
quetiapine (Seroquel) *or* aripiprazole (Abilify)	Schizophrenia	Drowsiness, decreased sweating, headache, nausea, vomiting	Weight gain, constipation	Neuroleptic malignant syndrome	Hypersensitivity
Atypical Antipsychotics *High Risk*					
clozapine (Clozaril)	Schizophrenia	Drowsiness, decreased sweating, headache, nausea, vomiting	Weight gain, constipation	Agranulocyto-sis (1%), seizures, myocarditis, lowering of pressure, Neuroleptic malignant syndrome, diabetes	Hypersensitivity

FIGURE 13: ANTIPSYCHOTIC MEDICATIONS: USES & RISKS

Adapted from BEFORE YOU TAKE THAT PILL, by J. Douglas Bremner, © 2008 J. Douglas Bremner, used by permission of Avery Publishing, an imprint of the Penguin Group.

Medications for the Treatment of Insomnia

These days not only are we sleepless in Seattle, we're having trouble getting some shut eye pretty much everywhere else as well. One in four busy Americans has some trouble sleeping, and many of them are taking prescription sleep medications or over-the-counter supplements. Sleep disturbances are of course a symptom of trauma-related mental disorders like PTSD and depression, of course, but many traumatized individuals can have sleep problems even in the absence of one of these diagnoses. Anti-insomnia medications may be helpful in the short term, but many patients will eventually need non-medication interventions for insomnia in the long run.

Insomnia can lead to a host of other problems. For instance, about 40% of people with insomnia also suffer from anxiety or depression. It is difficult to say whether the insomnia or the mental disorder comes first. Trouble falling and staying asleep can also affect memory and cognition and lead to obesity (alternatively obesity can impair sleep, e.g. in patients with sleep apnea).

In the past, barbiturate and benzodiazepine medications were the most common treatments of insomnia. Benzodiazepine medications, which are also used to treat anxiety, include:

- alprazolam (Xanax)

- clonazepam (Klonopin)

- temazepam (Restoril)

- triazolam (Halcion)

- oxazepam (Serax)

- lorazepam (Ativan)

- chlordiazepoxide (Librium)

- clorazepate (Tranxene)

- prazepam (Centrax)

- quazepam (Doral)

- estazolam (Prosom)

- diazepam (Valium)

- flurazepam (Dalmane)

Benzodiazepines all of the same mechanisms of action, binding to the GABA/benzodiazepine complex in the brain, resulting in release of the inhibitory neurotransmitter, GABA. The only difference between the different benzodiazepine medications is time to onset and duration of effect. On average, they make you fall asleep four minutes earlier and add an hour to your sleep time. Possible side effects that can occur the next day after taking these medications include:

- drowsiness

- dizziness

- light-headedness

- problems with memory

The benzodiazepines used to be in wide spread use amongst the elderly. The developer of the first medication in this class, diazepam (Valium), the Hoffmann-LaRoche Pharmaceutical Company, even pushed these medications for treatment of the general dreariness of being old, even though it is well documented that anxiety decreases and general life satisfaction increases with age. Subsequently it has been shown that benzodiazepines increase the risk of falling and getting a hip fracture in the elderly by 50%, and are associated with a 60% increase in road traffic accidents.

Because of these problems and concerns about the development of dependency with benzodiazepines alternatives for the treatment of insomnia were pursued. This led to the development of the "z" drugs, so-called because their generic names start with the letter z. One of these newer sleeping pills, zopiclone (Imovane), was like the benzodiazepines associated with an increased risk of road traffic accidents.

The z drugs include zaleplon (Sonata), zolpidem (Ambien), eszopiclone (Lunesta), and zopiclone (Imovane). These all act on specific subsets of the GABA receptor.

General side effects for all of these meds include:

- drowsiness

- memory impairment,

- headache

- dizziness

- nausea, and

- nervousness

The UK National Institute for Clinical Evidence (NICE) is an unbiased governmental body that provides information on clinical treatments based on reviews by their experts of the evidence. In a 2004 NICE review they reported that they found no difference between the different Z drugs (Sonata (zaleplon), Lunesta (eszopiclone), Ambien (zolpidem), or Imovane (zopiclone)) in efficacy, next-day impairment, or risk of withdrawal or dependence. As well, there were no benefits in terms of effectiveness or side effects compared to benzodiazepines. Recently reports have emerged of people doing strange things on these medications, like walking in their sleep, getting up to cook eggs or have sex, or even drive, and had absolutely no memory of it later. Combining these medications with alcohol seems to be particularly problematic.

Insomnia Medications: Risks and Benefits

Drug	Use	Common, benign side effects	Serious side effects	Life threatening side effects	Reasons not to take
Barbiturates *High Risk*					
phenobarbital (Luminal) *or* butabarbital (Butisol) *or* pentobarbital (Nembutal)	Insomnia	Drowsiness, lethargy, headache, dizziness	Problems breathing, delirium, depression	Allergic reaction, decreased blood counts (rare), respiratory depression, addiction	Allergy, addiction, depression
Antihistamines *Low Risk*					
hydroxyzine (Atarax, Vistaril)	Insomnia	Dry mouth, urinary retention	Confusion, night-mares, irritability	None	None
Benzodiazepines *Moderate Risk*					
alprazolam (Xanax) *or* clonazepam (Klonopin) *or* temazepam (Restoril) *or* oxazepam (Serax) *or* lorazepam (Ativan) *or* chlordiazepoxide (Librium) *or* clorazepate (Tranxene) *or* halazepam (Paxipam) *or*	Insomnia	Drowsiness	Dependency, memory loss, confusion	Hip fracture, driving accidents	History of addictions, memory impairment

Drug	Use	Common, benign side effects	Serious side effects	Life threatening side effects	Reasons not to take
prazepam (Centrax) *or* quazepam (Doral) *or* estazolam (Prosom) *or* diazepam (Valium) *or* flurazepam (Dalmane)					
triazolam (Halcion)	Insomnia	Drowsiness, early wake up	Dependency, memory loss, confusion	Hip fracture, driving accidents	History of addictions, memory impairment
Serotonin 1A Agonists *Low Risk*					
buspirone (Buspar)	Insomnia	Nausea, headache, light headedness	None	None	None
Z Drugs *Moderate Risk*					
zaleplon (Sonata) *or* zolpidem (Ambien) *or* zopiclone (Imovane)	Insomnia	Drowsiness, headache, nervousness	Memory loss	Sleep walking, driving accidents	Allergy to medication
eszopiclone (Lunesta)	Insomnia	Drowsiness, headache, nervousness, bad taste	Memory loss	Sleep walking, driving accidents	Allergy to medication
Melatonin Receptor Agonists *Low Risk*					
ramelteon	Insomnia	Headache,	diarrhea	depression	Pregnancy

Drug	Use	Common, benign side effects	Serious side effects	Life threatening side effects	Reasons not to take
(Rozerem)	a	drowsiness, fatigue, dizziness, nausea			or nursing

FIGURE 14: INSOMNIA MEDICATIONS: USES & RISKS

Adapted from BEFORE YOU TAKE THAT PILL, by J. Douglas Bremner, © 2008 J. Douglas Bremner, used by permission of Avery Publishing, an imprint of the Penguin Group.

In addition to these drugs, there are a handful of additional drugs that have sedative properties, and are prescribed and used "off label" for insomnia. These include drugs from allergy meds like antihistamines to antidepressants, some of which need a prescription and some can be bought in the pharmacy or "over the counter."

The most commonly prescribed antihistamine for insomnia is hydroxyzine (Atarax, Vistaril). Over-the-counter diphenhydramine (Benadryl, Simply Sleep, Tylenol PM, Excedrin PM and their "store brand" counterparts) are often recommended by doctors as sleep aids, and are effective for many people. These medications are relatively free of potential for addiction or abuse.

Side effects are less common than for the benzodiazepines or Z drugs and include:

- dry mouth and urinary retention

- irritability, and

- more rarely, confusion, nightmares, and nervousness

The most effective therapy for the treatment of insomnia has been shown in studies to be cognitive behavioral therapy, which works better than medication for sleeplessness and doesn't have any side effects. I'll cover CBT in the next chapter.

Stimulants

Doctors are increasingly diagnosing Attention Deficit Disorder (ADD) or Attention Deficit and Hyperactivity Disorder (ADHD) in adults, and the diagnosis in children is more common than it was several decades ago. ADD and ADHD are also seen more commonly in abused and neglected children. Whether the increase in diagnoses is due to an increase rate of the disorders or more awareness on the part of doctors is unclear. What is clear is that stimulants and similar medications are being used in increasing numbers. The most common ADHD drugs are methylphenidate (Ritalin), mixed amphetamine salts (Adderall), and atomoxetine (Strattera).

Ritalin (methylphenidate, Methylin) is a stimulant medication that works by increasing the release of dopamine in the brain. That helps you concentrate better. Ritalin can suppress growth slightly in children. Other side effects include: palpitations, nervousness, rapid heart rate, loss of appetite, increased blood pressure, headache, upset stomach, and mood changes. High doses can cause psychosis. Extended release forms of methylphenidate or drugs that are essentially identical include Concerta, Metadate, and dexmethylphenidate (Focalin). These drugs are essentially identical to Ritalin, and have no demonstrated difference in efficacy.

Another stimulant medication used in the treatment of ADHD is the amphetamine Adderall (mixed amphetamine salts). Adderall is a mixture of two forms of amphetamine, and is marketed as a medication that only has to be taken once a day. Dextroamphetamine (Dexedrine) is comprised of one of the forms of amphetamine but is essentially the same thing as Adderall. These drugs also work by increasing dopamine in the brain. Adderall can suppress your appetite, leading to weight loss. Like Ritalin, Adderall probably has some long-term growth suppression effects in kids. Other side effects are palpitations, nervousness, rapid heart rate, and upset stomach. Rarely there have been cases of cardiac arrest.

Another drug for the treatment of ADHD is atomoxetine (Strattera). Strattera blocks uptake of norepinephrine into the neuron. Strattera has the advantage over Adderall and Ritalin that it is not a stimulant and is therefore not associated with cardiac side effects. Side effects include indigestion, fatigue, dizziness, decreased appetite, and mood swings. Like Adderall, Strattera can inhibit growth in children.

Psychological treatments work better for some people than prescription medications (or helps augment the effects of than these medications). I cover this topic in the next chapter.

CHAPTER 9: PSYCHOLOGICAL THERAPY FOR TRAUMA

Psychological treatments have been shown to be useful for psychological trauma survivors with PTSD and depression and other trauma-related disorders.

Most psychological therapies involve some degree of mental exposure to the traumatic event in a safe, controlled environment, with an evaluation of their personal response to the exposure. This means the patient will be asked to recount the traumatic event, and talk about his thoughts, feelings, and cognitions about the event.

Examples of thoughts would be "I couldn't believe this was happening to me" or "my mother was just outside but I couldn't call out to her." Feelings would include anger, fear, disgust, and helplessness. Perceptions would include "I deserved this because I shouldn't have been there at that time."

Before starting therapy, important factors such as suicidality, substance abuse, panic, and disorganized thinking, must be evaluated and dealt with.

The next phase is educating both the patient, and the family and friends of the person affected, as discussed in more detail above.

Personally, I use either supportive or psychodynamic therapy with my trauma clients. I also give them a copy of my book *You Can't Just Snap Out of It*, which has workbooks and exercises that teach them ways to relax and cope with stress. I also tell patients that, for patients who are insightful and can tolerate therapy, it is ultimately the treatment of choice, although they may get worse before they get better, and it will take a lot longer than they thought and they will uncover more painful material than they thought. But that if they stick with it they will eventually feel better.

Many of the patients I see, especially in my clinic at the VA, are very fragile, and not able to tolerate intense therapy. Maybe they are unemployed, or are having trouble staying sober, or are homeless or have unstable living situations. The psychological trauma may be so overwhelming that they are not ready to deal with it. For them, supportive therapy, and possibly medications, is in order, just talking with them about their lives, educating them about symptoms, and helping them maintain control.

Cognitive Behavioral Therapy (CBT)

Cognitive Behavioral Therapy (CBT) involves a focus on the thoughts, feelings, and cognitions related to the traumatic event. It doesn't spend as much time talking about things not related to the trauma. CBT tries to correct negative or distorted thoughts or cognitions about the actual trauma.

Many CBT therapists evaluate levels of distress using something like the Subjective Units of Distress Scale (SUDS). The SUDS asks how distressed the client is feeling at the time on a scale of 0 (not distressed at all) to 100 (extremely distressed). Therapists will typically administer the SUDS at the beginning and end of a therapy session, and after going through evoking imagery of a traumatic event.

Specifics of the CBT technique involve taking one element of the trauma at a time (known as "desensitization") so that the traumatic event is not too overwhelming.

Most therapists also teach relaxation techniques (deep breathing, muscle stretching, and relaxation) to help clients get through the imagery of a traumatic memory. I talk more about these techniques in Chapter 10, "Tools for Coping with Stress."

Another technique involves developing a mental image in the mind of a safe and happy place...maybe a place on the beach, or up on a mountain top. First the client develops the image of that place so they can quickly return to it. Then if they get too overwhelmed with traumatic images, they can switch to the safe place to bring down their anxiety level.

The therapist will then discuss the traumatic event and try and elicit all of the sensations associated with it. What did the client see, hear, smell, touch, and what were the feelings associated with it. Sometimes clients have trouble identifying emotions, in which case you might want to show them a printout of the list of emotional words listed in an appendix of this book. You can also print out the words from my web site at startnowprogram.com.

Traumatic experiences are often experienced in a distorted way. Cognitions about the event may be incorrect, and part of the therapy involves correcting these perceptions. There are often gaps or jumps in the memory, including episodes of dissociative amnesia. The inchoate nature of the traumatic event may be a barrier to recovery. Fragments of the event came back at inopportune times, create anxiety and make the traumatized individual feel out of control. I have found that encouraging clients to write, paint, or draw their experiences can help to create a cohesive narrative. Another technique is to have the client return to the scene of an accident and get an accurate, non-trauma-related view of the place. We outline these techniques in the book written for clients called *You Just Can't Snap Out of It.* Some of the workbooks in the book are also on our website and can be downloaded for free at startnowprogram.com. Creating a cohesive narrative with correct cognitions is actually part of the therapeutic process.

In CBT, exposure to the imagery of the traumatic event occurs repeatedly over the course of the sessions, with administration of the SUDS, to show a decrease in distress related to the traumatic images. Sometimes therapists will ask clients to do "homework" where the images are invoked at home and the clients do their own self ratings. Exposure therapy is usually pretty effective if people can stick with it, but many trauma survivors cannot tolerate it and drop out of treatment.

Cognitive Behavioral Therapy for the Treatment of Insomnia

As I pointed out in the last chapter, cognitive behavioral therapy is also useful in the treatment of insomnia. CBT for insomnia involves replacing negative cognitions and unrealistic expectations about sleep with more helpful ones, and in changing behavioral routines that interfere with sleep.

The first step is to replace negative thoughts ("I can't sleep without medications") with more positive ones ("If I take the time to relax, I can get to sleep without help from pills.") The underlying theory is that one should "retrain" their brain to learn to sleep peacefully and deeply again.

Changing sleep habits is the second piece of cognitive therapy. For example,

- using the bed and bedroom only for sleep (no working or TV-watching in bed; insomniacs often spend too much time in bed trying to sleep, and the best thing to do is to get out of bed and read for a while or listen to soft music),

- setting and maintaining a regular sleep schedule,

- eliminating daytime naps,

- minimizing or avoiding altogether caffeine, alcohol, stimulants, and heavy or extremely spicy meals four to six hours before going to bed, and

- relaxation techniques such as progressive muscle relaxation often help. It involves alternately contracting individual muscles and relaxing with exhalation; the individual goes progressively through the body one muscle group at a time.

Behavioral changes are highly effective, and, best of all, persist for a longer period of time than drug therapy. About 80% of patients will show improvement. The time to fall asleep is reduced from sixty-five minutes to thirty-five minutes, an increase in sleep time of thirty minutes, and improved subjective ratings of sleep quality.

Since long-term use of sleeping pills is not recommended, people with chronic insomnia really need to make the effort to get sleep behavioral therapy treatment, or, at a minimum, educate themselves through reading or online about the principles promoted in CBT programs for insomnia.

Meditation and gentle yoga can also help some people fall asleep more easily as part of a cognitive therapy program or on their own.

Systematic Desensitization and Imaginal Exposure Therapies

Two techniques closely related to CBT and often used together include systematic desensitization and imaginal exposure therapies.

In systematic desensitization, there is pairing of a reminder of the trauma with relaxation, so that the anxiety associated with thinking about the traumatic event is inhibited by relaxation. When the client becomes anxious, they are instructed to erase the scene, relax, and then imagine the scenario again. This is repeated until anxiety is no longer associated with the imagination.

In imaginal exposure therapy, the client is asked to imagine the event in their mind and focus on thoughts and emotions as if the event were happening now. Instructions for imaginal therapy might go something like this:

- I want you to close your eyes and begin to talk about the assault.

- Talk about it in the first person, as if it is happening to you right now.

- As you're talking, picture the story in your mind, and describe what is happening.

- Describe it in as much detail as possible, including what you're doing, what he's doing, what you're thinking and feeling.

- Try not to let go of the image, even if it's upsetting to you, and

- We will talk about it after the exposure is finished.

Other treatments effective for PTSD fall into the category of anxiety management, which are discussed next.

Stress Inoculation Training (SIT)

Stress Inoculation Training (SIT) involves several anxiety-management techniques, including:

- psychoeducation

- muscle relaxation training

- breathing retraining

- role playing

- covert modeling

- guided self-dialogue

- thought stopping

This treatment program has been shown to be effective in the treatment of PTSD.

Eye Movement Desensitization and Reprocessing (EMDR) Therapy

Another type of therapy that has been shown to work is Eye Movement Desensitization and Reprocessing (EMDR) therapy.

This involves having patients follow a moving finger while visualizing their trauma. Newer versions of EMDR have involved other methods like tapping on alternative shoulders during re-exposure to the trauma. Controlled studies have shown the usefulness of this technique for treating trauma.

Hypnosis in the Treatment of Psychological Trauma

Although hypnosis has had a controversial place in the treatment of stress-related psychiatric disorders, in the hands of competent and trained professionals, it does serve a potentially useful role.

Memories not available to consciousness due to processes such as dissociative amnesia may be accessed through hypnosis. Some studies have shown that hypnosis may lead to an improvement in PTSD symptoms.

When memories that were not previously fully available are brought into consciousness, they can be processed for the emotional and cognitive content, and gradually integrated into the patient's normal storehouse of memories.

This process must be performed with caution because the reintroduction of traumatic memories into consciousness may be associated with a feeling of upset and an increase in psychiatric symptoms. Some therapists get written informed consent from patients who are to undergo hypnosis, so that these patients can recognize the potential limitations and pitfalls.

Psychodynamic Therapy

Although psychodynamic therapy has not been subjected to as much research, it clearly is useful for many survivors of psychological trauma. Psychologically-oriented or psychodynamic therapy typically involves meeting one-on-one with a therapist for once a week and talking about things related to the trauma, as well as things in the here and now and how they are connected to the original trauma. It also involves evaluating the thoughts and feelings the client develops about the therapist and the therapy itself. The course of therapy is typically much longer than for CBT, extending weeks and sometimes years.

Psychodynamic therapy helps trauma patients understand what the meaning of their trauma is for them as human beings. It also involves a lot of the techniques involved in the therapies listed above, like examining the basis in reality for a lot of the cognitions related to the trauma, or anxiety related to memories of the trauma.

Group Therapy

Our guess is that you won't find many people in therapy groups who will tell your clients to just get over it or to just snap out of it.

Groups are best when they are led by two mental health professionals with training and experience in running group therapy.

Making the Connection

Different therapists have different orientations, but successful therapists all share in common a commitment to, and belief in, their methods, and a professional and empathic approach to their clients. Studies have shown that the ability of the therapist and the individual fit with the client, and the belief that the therapist has in the value of the treatment, are more important than which of many theoretical orientations are used.

Therapy can help in many ways, from learning a feeling of safety, getting validation for one's self as a person and appreciating the magnitude of the psychological trauma that has been experienced, to getting grounded within a crazy-making family.

In psychological therapies the client talks about how they relate to the therapist. By getting honest and unbiased feedback from a neutral source, the client learns how they relate to other people in their life, and how the trauma has affected those interactions. The therapist may be the first person a trauma victim has talked to about certain experiences, and may be the first to not respond with comments like "just get over it," "snap out of it," or "move on."

How Therapy Works on the Brain

Psychological therapies are probably effective because of the way they act on the brain to reverse the effects of trauma. As discussed above, one of the hallmarks of psychological trauma is an inability to extinguish fear responses with reminders of the trauma. In full-blown PTSD patients, this can become very disabling, to the point where it interferes with daily activities. For these patients, dysfunction in the prefrontal cortex leads to an inability to extinguish traumatic memories through inhibition of activity in the amygdala. One of the roles of these therapies is to help the brain to inhibit or extinguish traumatic memories through techniques such as gradual exposure to traumatic reminders in the supportive context of therapy, also known as "desensitization."

I discussed above the laboratory model of conditioned fear responses, how pairing an unconditioned stimulus (e.g., an electric shock) with a conditioned stimulus (e.g., bright light) leads to a fear reaction to the conditioned stimulus ("bright light") alone. With repeated exposure to the conditioned stimulus, there is a decrease in fear responding, related to an inhibition of the amygdala (which plays a critical role in learning fear) by the prefrontal cortex.

In a similar way in normal individuals, fear responses to reminders of the trauma normally become extinguished with repeated exposure to reminders of the trauma. However, for PTSD patients, dysfunction in the prefrontal cortex leads to an inability to extinguish traumatic memories through inhibition of activity in the amygdala.

One of the roles of behavioral therapies is to facilitate the ability of the brain to inhibit or extinguish traumatic memories, through techniques such as gradual exposure to traumatic reminders, in the supportive context of a therapeutic environment.

Getting Help For Clients With Limited Means

Since PTSD or depression related to trauma can affect the ability of clients to work, many trauma patients have difficulty paying for treatment. If your client cannot afford to go to see a medical doctor or psychiatrist, here are some other options:

- Psychiatrists can get free samples of one of the newer antidepressants from pharmaceutical sales representatives.

- Some of the drug companies have compassionate care programs your client can sign up for to get free medications. Part of the application may need to be filled out by a psychiatrist.

- Finally, your client can get a generic version of an antidepressant and buy it at Walmart for about $44.00 a month. There are other discount deals available at other stores they might want to keep an eye out for.

- If your client has trouble sleeping there are over-the-counter medications I talked about in the prior chapter like diphenhydramine (Benadryl).

- They can also do things like exercise, which is free and helps mental symptoms.

Finally, you can point your clients to our free START-NOW program workbook. They can also download the workbook for free from http://www.dougbremner.com/startnowworkbook.pdf.

The Bottom Line for the Treatment of Trauma

The bottom line is that for clients with psychological trauma and the diagnosis of depression or PTSD, psychotherapy is the treatment of choice, if they can tolerate it, are financially stable, not actively abusing drugs or alcohol, and have enough intelligence and insight to benefit. For those who are too emotionally fragile (which may be the majority), the treatment of choice is supportive psychotherapy, where the goal is to not talk about the trauma, but to help shore up the client's defense mechanisms so they can function. These patients may eventually graduate to a more insight-oriented therapy. Medication should also be considered as an adjunct to treatment, possibly by getting a consultation with a psychiatrist.

The message from research on treatments for the mental health effects of psychological trauma and the effects of psychological trauma on the brain is that there is hope. Symptoms related to trauma are mediated by the brain. If we can reverse these brain changes, we can reverse the symptoms. Clients should be encouraged to take an active role in their recovery. They can do this by following the steps in the workbook linked to above, engaging in psychotherapy, possibly adding medication, improving diet and lifestyle, and by learning tools for coping with stress, which I discuss in the next chapter.

CHAPTER 10: TOOLS FOR COPING WITH STRESS

This chapter covers tools for coping with stress that you can teach to your clients. They're free, they usually don't have side effects, and clients can do them on their own time. Most mental health clinicians will already be familiar with these tools, but they are included here for completeness and as a checklist for topics to cover with your clients. Also, specific images can be used as a guide, and instructions to all of these exercises are on our website startnowprogram.com, so you can print them out for your clients. This material is also in the book written for victims of psychological trauma, *You Can't Just Snap Out Of It,"* which they can get on amazon.com

Deep Breathing

One tool for coping with stress which clients can do on their own or with your help is deep breathing. Here are some simple instructions you can give your client (you can print out the instructions on startnowprogram.com.

1. Sit comfortably with your back straight. If you feel more comfortable that way, lie on the floor.

2. Put one hand on your chest and the other on your stomach.

3. Focus on your breath going in and out of your body.

4. Breathe deeply from your stomach, rather than taking shallow breaths in your chest, getting as much fresh air as possible in your lungs. This will get more oxygen into

your lungs, which will make you feel less tense, short of breath, and anxious.

5. Now breathe in through your nose.

The hand on your stomach should rise, while the hand on your chest doesn't move much. If you are lying on the floor, you can put something on your stomach and watch it rise and fall.

6. Breathe out through your mouth, pushing out as much air as you can while squeezing your stomach muscles. The hand on your stomach should move in as you breathe out, but your other hand shouldn't move much.

7. Continue to breathe in through your nose and out through your mouth.

8. Try to inhale enough so that your stomach rises and falls.

9. Count slowly as you exhale.

Progressive Muscle Relaxation

Progressive muscle relaxation involves progressively moving through one's body and tensing and relaxing all of the muscles. This helps clients learn where their body carries stress. Instruct clients to lie on the floor and take off their shoes, or if in a public place, to do it while sitting:

1. Start at your feet and move your way up your body.

2. Take a deep breath and hold it.

3. Push your toes down like you are stepping on the gas as hard as you can for five seconds.

4. Now slowly relax your muscles as you let your breath leave your body.

5. Breathe out.

6. Sit there for a few seconds breathing in and out while focusing on your body and how it feels.

7. Now, pull your toes up toward your nose as hard as you can.

8. Breathe out.

9. Continue to breathe in with muscle tightening and out with relaxing with short resting periods after relaxing.

10. Tighten the muscles in your calves. Breathe in. Relax your muscles. Breathe out.

11. Now tighten the muscles the ones in your thighs. Breathe in. Relax your muscles. Breathe out.

12. Tighten the muscles in your buttocks. Breathe in. Relax your muscles. Breathe out.

13. Tighten your stomach muscles. Breathe in. Relax your muscles. Breathe out.

14. Scrunch your shoulders up toward your head. Breathe in. Relax your muscles. Breathe out.

15. Squeeze your hands. Breathe in. Relax your muscles. Breathe out.

16. Pull your hands up to your shoulders. Breathe in. Relax your muscles. Breathe out.

17. Now stretch your arms out straight. Breathe in. Relax your muscles. Breathe out.

18. Pull your head down to your chest. Breathe in. Relax your muscles. Breathe out.

19. Push your head to the right, all the way until it is tight. Breathe in. Relax your muscles. Breathe out.

20. Push your head to the left. Breathe in. Relax your muscles. Breathe out.

21. Now go through the different muscle groups in your face, one-by-one.

Tell clients that when they are done they should remain silent and focus on their breath going in and out for three minutes. As they breathe they can feel the tension leave their bodies every time they breathe out. If they want they can visualize a peaceful scene on the beach or in the mountains.

Guided Visual Imagery

Another technique to help your client cope with stress is guided visual imagery. Guided visual imagery involves imagining a peaceful scene where one can let go of stress. Instruct clients to think of a place they have been or make up something new in their mind. It might be a tropical beach, a place in the mountains, or a place they used to go to be alone and feel safe when they were children. Tell them to close their eyes so they can bring the scene into their mind.

For instance, say your client sees herself in an alpine meadow. The sky is blue with a few wispy white clouds in the sky. The grey granite of rocky peaks rises all around. There is a slight breeze and the lazy buzzing of some insects far away. The short green alpine grass and yellow and white alpine flowers rustle in the breeze. You can suggest to her that she is all alone. Tell her to feel the wind slightly rustling her hair and the sun upon her cheek. Have her picture the mountain scene or wherever she has decided to go as vividly as possible. Tell her to see the colors, smell the smells, hear the sounds, and feel the sensations of the scene. Tell her to try and bring in as many sensory processes as possible. As she visualizes the scene, tell her to focus on her breathing, and feel her stress and worries slip away.

Mindful Meditation

Mindful meditation is rapidly growing in popularity as a tool for coping with stress.

In our research studies, we have found mindful meditation to be an effective treatment for PTSD, both in Iraq vets as well as PTSD related to other traumas. It also reverses some of the changes in the brain associated with trauma. Mindful meditation incorporates some of the tools mentioned above, including focusing on the breath and the body. Mindfulness involves being fully present in the current time and letting thoughts about the future and the past slip away.

The process involves a detached awareness of one's own thoughts and breathing without being overly critical of one's own thoughts or over-thinking an experience. If a judgmental thought about anxiety or stress reactions or behavior comes into your client's mind, instruct them to not fight it, just note it and then let it move away.

Mindfulness is useful because it removes the process of dwelling on the past, on thinking about things we could have done, or worrying about what will happen in the future. That is because there is nothing we can do to change the past, and in the vast majority of cases, little we can do to change the future. We waste an inordinate amount of time thinking about these things, which raises our stress levels. Mindfulness is a way of teaching oneself to focus on what is happening right now

In the body scan, the client is instructed to focus attention on various parts of the body. Like for progressive muscle relaxation, instruct your client to start with the feet and work their way up. However, instead of tensing and relaxing the muscles, they should simply focus on the way each part of their body feels, without labeling the sensations as either "good" or "bad."

You don't have to be seated or still to meditate. In walking meditation, mindfulness involves being focused on the physicality of each step — the sensation of your feet touching the ground, the rhythm of your breath while moving, and feeling the wind against your face.

A related area is mindful eating. For your clients who have problems with over-eating or using food to regulate their mood, instruct them to sit at the table and focus their full attention on the meal (no TV, newspapers, or eating on the run). Tell them to eat slowly, taking the time to fully enjoy and concentrate on each bite. We can learn something from the Slow Food movement in Italy.

Mindfulness meditation is not equal to zoning out. It takes effort to maintain concentration and to bring it back to the present moment when the mind wanders. Mindfulness meditation actually changes the brain, strengthening the areas associated with joy and relaxation, and weakening those involved in negativity and stress.

You can help your client in your sessions, or refer them to classes that are taught now throughout the country by "teachers" certified by the Center for Mindfulness at the Massachusetts Medical School in Worcester, Massachusetts.

Print out the instructions for the tools for coping with stress and give them to your clients!

CHAPTER 11: BETTER LIFESTYLES AS A TOOL FOR RECOVERY FROM PSYCHOLOGICAL TRAUMA

Making changes in diet and lifestyle is an important part of recovery from psychological trauma. Not only does this improve physical health, it also will benefit your client's mental health as well.

Eating right, exercising, and changing other aspects of lifestyle can affect how you feel, and how you feel about yourself. Making these changes has also been shown to be useful in the treatment of mental disorders, like depression and PTSD.

Psychological Trauma Can Affect both Physical and Mental Health

People with a history of psychological trauma have a number of strikes against them when it comes to health. For starters, trauma leads to an increase in risky behaviors that threaten good health. For instance, women with a history of childhood sexual abuse have been shown to have an increase in obesity.

Childhood trauma is also associated with an increase in smoking, using drugs, using too many prescription medications like sedatives and pain killers, and drinking too much alcohol. Childhood trauma, especially child sexual abuse in women, leads to an increase in unsafe sex, number of sexual encounters and multiple partners, although interestingly there is a decrease in sexual satisfaction.

Dr. Rob Anda, a doctor and scientist we collaborate with at the Centers for Disease Control (CDC) (it's right next door to Emory University, where we work and have our Clinical Neuroscience Research Unit (ECNRU), in Atlanta, Georgia), did a study that showed that childhood trauma increased the risk for intravenous drug abuse by *ten-fold!* That's a greater risk than getting lung cancer from smoking.

Benefits of Exercise for Trauma Victims

Exercise helps trauma victims in more ways than one. Not only does it improve physical health, it is also good for mental health. The best way to burn off energy from the "fight or flight" response and elevated stress hormones is exercise.

How much should you advise your clients to exercise?

I recommend that trauma survivors exercise at least three times a week for thirty minutes. If they don't want to run, however, they can go for a brisk walk. Even that counts as exercise.

Studies have shown that exercise is an excellent treatment for mental disorders like depression and PTSD. In fact, exercise is as good as Zoloft (sertraline) for depression! Other studies showed that exercise works as well as antidepressants for the treatment of PTSD. Even just a few hours of walking per week helps. Exercise results in increased vitality and life satisfaction, and decreased levels of stress. Exercise results in a surge of serotonin, the neurotransmitter which make us feel good right, after working out, as well as a long-term mood shift after regular exercise is established.

Exercise also has positive effects on the brain, reversing the effects of trauma. Exercise results in increased growth in brain cells in the hippocampus, the opposite of the effects of stress. This is a good non-chemical way for your client to restore their brains to the condition it was prior to their trauma. Regular exercise has favorable effects on the immune system as well, which may promote health, especially for people who are stressed and/or depressed.

Exercise is far less expensive, and more easily accessible, than medication and psychotherapy. Plus, it has none of the side effects, such as sexual dysfunction, as seen with some antidepressants. Indeed, the "side effects" of using exercise as an antidepressant are beneficial to general well-being:

- improved heart health,

- increased strength,

- lessening depression and anxiety, and

- weight loss.

Healthy Eating

Healthy eating is another crucial part of your client's better lifestyles program. I think people should cook their own food, because that is the best way to have fresh and healthy ingredients and avoid preservatives. Making your own meals is also essential to making sure that you eat a lot of fruits and vegetables, which are key to good health.

People who are depressed and/or have a history of childhood psychological trauma have an increase in risk for obesity as adults. Eating diets high in fat can interfere with the formation of serotonin, a neurotransmitter implicated in depression, which might affect mood.

Studies have also shown that ingestion of fat results in a temporary drop in mood. Remember the guy from the movie *Super Size Me*, Morgan Spurlock? He was practically psycho after a month of eating nothing but McDonald's food.

It is important for your clients to learn how to cook, so that they can stay away from fast food restaurants, where they are almost sure to get too much fat and too many calories, and not enough of the things needed for good health like fresh fruits and vegetables. Relying on fast food restaurants and eating a poor diet will increases weight and has a negative effect on mood. That in turn will is a barrier to recovery from psychological trauma.

A long time ago people noticed that people from Italy live longer and seemed to get less disease than people in the U.S. This led to the idea that maybe something about differences in diet, which came to be known as the Mediterranean Diet, could account for this.

The Mediterranean Diet is associated with sustained weight loss. This diet is:

• high in vegetables, legumes, fruits, nuts, cereals, and fish,

• low in meat and poultry and dairy products,

• recommended alcohol consumption of ten to 50 grams (1-4 glasses of wine) per day for men, and five to twenty-five grams (1-2 glasses of wine) for women

• The diet substitutes unsaturated fats (olive oil) for saturated and monounsaturated fats (butter, animal fat).

The Mediterranean Diet:

• reduces heart disease, stroke, diabetes, and cancer risk,

• prolongs life (following the Mediterranean Diet is associated with a reduction in mortality by one half over a four-year time period in some populations),

• cuts the number of heart attacks in half in patients with heart disease, an effect that in one study was twice as good as medication treatment.

• Overall, the effects of these diets were superior to medications for weight loss and the prevention of heart disease and diabetes, with fewer side effects and more positive effects on well-being.

See the figure below, provided courtesy of Oldways Preservation and Exchange Trust, a nonprofit foundation dedicated to promotion of the Mediterranean Diet and other healthy behaviors. Diet modifications including following the Mediterranean Diet have been shown to have a protective effect against the development of several neurological disorders, including Parkinson's Disease (PD), Multiple Sclerosis, Mild Cognitive Impairment (MCI) and Alzheimer's Disease.

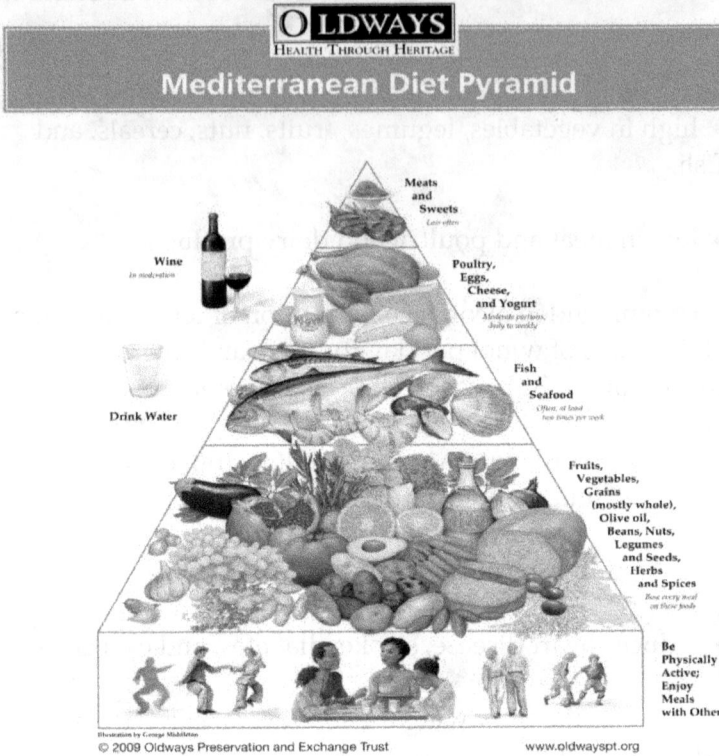

OLDWAYS
HEALTH THROUGH HERITAGE

Mediterranean Diet Pyramid

Meats
and
Sweets
Less often

Wine
in moderation

Poultry,
Eggs,
Cheese,
and Yogurt
*Moderate portions,
daily to weekly*

Fish
and
Seafood
*Often, at least
two times per week*

Drink Water

Fruits,
Vegetables,
Grains
(mostly whole),
Olive oil,
Beans, Nuts,
Legumes
and Seeds,
Herbs
and Spices
*Base every meal
on these foods*

Be
Physically
Active;
Enjoy
Meals
with Others

Illustration by George Middleton

© 2009 Oldways Preservation and Exchange Trust   www.oldwayspt.org

MEDITERRANEAN
FOODS · ALLIANCE
AN OLDWAYS PROGRAM

FIGURE 15: MEDITERRANEAN DIET FOOD PYRAMID
The diet is high in olive oil, fish, nuts, and breads, and low in red meat.
Figure courtesy of Oldways Preservation and Exchange Trust.
http://oldwayspt.org/resources/heritage-pyramids/mediterranean-diet-pyramid Copyright   © 2012 Oldways Preservation and Exchange Trust, used with permission.

Adding folate to the diet (associated with a reduction in homocysteine in the blood) helps with symptoms of depression, and at least one study showed that taking omega-3 fatty acid supplements helped symptoms of bipolar disorder.

Symptoms of Alcohol and Substance Abuse and Dependence
• Arrest for Driving Under the Influence (DUI)
• Missing days at work or being late to work because of drug or alcohol abuse
• Needing increasingly larger amounts of the substance for the same effect
• Trying to cut down but not being able to
• Being told repeatedly by friends and family that your drug or alcohol abuse is a problem
• Getting into accidents or sustaining injuries as a result of drug or alcohol abuse
• Not being able to remember what happened or having blackouts during drinking or drug use

FIGURE 16: SYMPTOMS OF ALCOHOL AND SUBSTANCE ABUSE

Getting Substance Abuse Under Control

Many survivors of psychological trauma use alcohol to reduce their anxiety and stress symptoms.

A history of arrest for Driving Under the Influence (DUI) is often good evidence that someone's drinking is out of control. Getting into an accident, being late for work, missing work, or getting into trouble at work because of drinking or using drugs are also indicators of a problem. Being often told by friends and family that your drinking or substance use is a problem should be taken as a warning sign. Clients cannot benefit from therapy if their minds are clouded by drugs and alcohol, so they have to get those problems under control.

The Risks of Prescription Drugs

Although some prescription medications are often helpful for trauma-related mental conditions, others can be a problem, or mixing them with alcohol or drugs can have dangerous effects. More people die in the U.S. every year now from overdoses of prescription medications (usually sleeping pills, sedatives, and pain meds) than from illegal drugs or car accidents. Big offenders are the pain medication oxycodone, and benzodiazepines like Valium (Diazepam) and Xanax (Alprazolam).

Who are these people that are dying from prescription drugs?

More than half of all Americans are now on at least one prescription drug, and 81% take some kind of pill. We spend twice as much money on drugs, and take twice as many drugs as other countries, but still our healthcare outcomes are second to last amongst industrialized countries. Even England is better, even though the English have a worse diet, and smoke and drink more than Americans.

As discussed in my book, *Before You Take That Pill: Why the Drug Industry May Be Bad For Your Health: Risks and Side Effects You Won't Find on the Label of Commonly Prescribed Drugs, Vitamins and Supplements,* (published by Penguin Press in 2008), studies show that for many conditions, including heart disease and diabetes, making changes in diet and lifestyle are often better than taking prescription medications.

The Bottom Line on Better Lifestyles

I recommend that clients with psychological trauma cook most of their own meals, eat fish twice a week, drink water instead of soda, use a lot of olive oil, eat a lot of fresh fruit and vegetables, add nuts to their dishes, and exercise three times a week, even if it is just taking long walks.

These changes will not only improve physical health, they will reduce stress-related symptoms, symptoms of depression and PTSD, and help burn off extra fight or flight energy that are a by-product of psychological trauma.

CHAPTER 12: WORKING TOGETHER AS COUPLES

Psychological trauma affects not only the individuals who are exposed to trauma, but also intimate partners closest to them. Working with the partners of clients with a history of psychological trauma can be a powerful tool in recovery.

Intimate partners are a critical component of recovery from psychological trauma. That's why I think it is so important to make the bond between couples stronger — to help them on their joint path toward recovery from psychological trauma.

Effects of Psychological Trauma on Relationships

Traumatic stress can take a big hit on relationships. Avoidance, retreat from other people, emotional numbing, and irritability can introduce problems into any relationship, and these are all behaviors that are closely linked to psychological trauma. If someone has PTSD and/or depression, the problem is even worse.

This is unfortunate, since the most important thing in recovery from psychological trauma is to have the love and support of a partner. When your traumatized clients are under siege, they need close and supportive relationships

How Do You Make Great Relationships?

How do you strengthen relationships? Everyone assumes that they know how to "do" relationships with others. But is that really the case?

Not really. You can teach clients how to have great relationships, just like you can teach someone to ride a bicycle. For survivors of psychological trauma, it's even more important.

So what makes for a great relationship?

The most important things are honesty, trust, equality, respect, mutual support, shared goals, flexibility, and friendship. While these things are important for everyone, they are especially important for psychological trauma survivors.

Sharing With a Partner Promotes Greater Intimacy

Your traumatized clients should be helped to learn when and where they share sensitive personal information. There are many situations, e.g. with unhelpful family members, where it is not a good idea to share. They do, however, need to find someone they can trust, and that person is usually an intimate partner.

Couples need to share thoughts and feelings openly. The more they can share about thoughts and feelings with their partner, the greater intimacy they will have in their relationships.

Building Trust

The foundation of every relationship is trust. For psychological trauma survivors who have had their trust violated, learning to trust again, this is even more important. It takes time and effort to build up the trust in a partnership or marriage and maintain it.

Open communication is healthy. Your clients should understand that communicating with their partner is critical. They shouldn't hold back the bad stuff in an effort to protect them. Your partner wants to hear from you, if it's bad news. Sharing both the good and the bad deepens the sense of intimacy. Caring for someone who is sick, wounded, or in a vulnerable position makes the bond stronger.

We want to be connected!

Sharing Equal Roles in a Relationship

It is critical that the two persons in a partnership have equal roles. One person may bring home the big paycheck, and the other one is a stay-at-home mom without an income, but the different roles should be seen as equal. Taking care of the children is not less important than working in a job for pay. Partners must work together as a team, make decisions together and have equal input, whether it is about money, children, or other issues.

Have Common Dreams

Clients should be taught to share common dreams with their partner. Couples that dream together grow together and stay together. They should be talking with their partners about the following things:

- When do you want to retire?

- Where?

- What kind of aspirations do you have for your kids?

- Do you want them to have the opportunity to go to college?

These are all things that need to be discussed early on and openly. Working at cross purposes with your partner can be exhausting. So don't do it!

The Importance of Shared Goals

Related to having shared dreams is having shared goals. It is important for couples to explicitly outline their goals and come to an agreement about them. Make a list of what they would like to accomplish together:

- Where do you want to live?

- Does a big house matter to you?

- How many kids do you want?

- What would you like for them to accomplish?

It's also important to be ready to revise family goals when needed. To do that, your clients will need to have frank and open discussions with their partner on a regular basis.

Having shared experiences builds trust and makes for stronger bonds. Encourage your clients to try and find fun things to do with their partner. They should have a store of positive memories for the bad times. Tell them to find ten minutes at the end of the day to catch up on what happened in the other partner's day. Find time away from work, kids, and other family to sit down and have an open and honest conversation. Go out on a date.

Flexibility in the Marriage

To make a marriage work, it is important to be flexible. Life doesn't always go according to plan. Couples need to be ready to adjust when things go wrong -- and they will! The key ingredient to marital success is the willingness of both partners to work together to overcome the problems that will inevitably arise.

Clients should be advised not to try and change their partner. Often when there is a history of psychological trauma there is attendant alcoholism or other addictions, or a history of violence. Sometimes people marry someone hoping they can fix them after the marriage. That never works. The truth is most us won't change. Advise them to learn to accept their partner as he or she is.

Having a Family

A past history of psychological trauma can have an impact on the family. Many people who have had a traumatic childhood are hesitant to have kids of their own, because they don't want to bring children into a cruel world, or they don't want to take the chance that their children will suffer. Maybe they feel they don't have a good handle on their emotions, or that, because of learned patterns from childhood, they may perpetuate the abuse they experienced as children onto their own children. In my clinical experience, this is indeed a common pattern in those who do not grapple with the demons of their past through therapy.

Having children can be a positive experience, however, for survivors of psychological trauma. Raising children can be a positive corrective experience, as they provide a better and safer environment for their children, and come to realize the positive emotional factors involved in having a family (as opposed to the negative experiences from their own childhood). A supportive family is a rich source of meaning, love, and connection. Clients should be advised, however, to be mindful about how their trauma might impact on their ability to work together with their partner as co-parents.

Traps and Pitfalls in the Marriage Relationship

There are a number of traps people can fall into in a marriage, and some of them are specific to couples where one or both partners are affected by psychological trauma:

- As I said before, one trap people get into is thinking that they will "fix" their partner after they marry them. They might use wishful thinking, with the idea that marriage will help their partner change. People should go into a marriage with the attitude that what you see is what you get.

- Another way people try to fix their marriage is by having kids. Many trauma survivors may feel a lack of connection with their partner or a personal inner void. They think that bringing a child into their lives will fill the void, or improve the connection with the spouse. Although children can enrich our lives, this shouldn't be the reason for your clients to have them. That just creates a situation where children come into the world already loaded with excess baggage.

- Marriages where one partner is a trauma victim and lead to rescue fantasies, where one partner wants to save the other. Although the marriage connection can help personal growth, this shouldn't be the reason for the marriage, because it creates an unstable foundation that may not withstand the rocky shoals that all marriages eventually encounter.

- Another trap is the attitude that someone is going to stay in a no matter what. This might come from beliefs based on one's church or background, or the concern that divorce will harm the children. Usually if the parents are fighting the children are relieved when they separate, as they don't have to be put in the uncomfortable position of choosing sides.

- In a related way, sacrificing everything for the children is another potential marriage trap, letting your marriage take a back seat to your children. This rarely achieves the purported goal, which is to help the children, and can lead to damage to the marriage. Putting too much emphasis on the kids may be an unconscious attempt to avoid the elephant in the room, which is the psychological trauma that one of the partners was exposed to. Your clients and their partners need to support each other's needs as adults to have the right mental state to be good parents.

Sexual Relations are an Important Part of Intimacy

Sometimes with everything taking up your client's time and energy, sexual relations with their partner may go on the back burner. Intrusive memories or complex emotions related to childhood sexual abuse can also interfere with one's sex life. Medical or psychiatric problems can also interfere. Or they may be on an antidepressant that has low libido as a side effect.

An active sex life, however, is a critical part of any relationship. It is the glue that holds the relationship together. Couples should be encouraged to talk about their sex lives openly. Sunlight is the best disinfectant, even if it can feel awkward or strange to talk about such private matters.

Raising Kids

One of the biggest causes of stress and conflict in marriages are arguments about how to raise the children. It is important that a couple agrees on how to parent their kids. They need to approach children as a team. Your clients should be encouraged to meet with their spouse apart from their children and agree on what kind of rules and boundaries they want for them. There will not always be complete agreement, but these differences of opinion need to be ironed out away from the children. They should not be witnesses to a public debate about what is the best way to set limits for them.

Another pitfall is allying with one or more children against the partner. This kind of dysfunctional behavior could have been learned in the family of origin that was the source of the original trauma. This splitting behavior, however, can be quite damaging to a marriage.

Money is a Major Source of Stress in Marriages

The other major stress in marriages is conflicts over money. Partners in a couple often have different approaches to saving and spending money. Imbalances in income levels can be a stressor, and if one or the other partner accumulates a lot debt that can intrude into the relationship. Couples should be encouraged to talk openly about money. There should be no financial secrets in a marriage, otherwise things will go awry. Couples need to find a way to compromise so both partners feel satisfied with the approach to finances. They should be making financial decisions as a team.

Bottom Line for Couples

In summary, couples should be encouraged to keep all lines of communication open. They should watch out for critical issues around raising children and money that can bring a marriage down. Staying committed and monogamous helps build trust and provides a solid foundation for the marriage.

Couples should be encouraged to have fun together, talk to each other, and spend time alone as a couple. They should work as partners in parenting children. And when all else fails, they need to learn how to say "I'm sorry."

CHAPTER 13: MILITARY FAMILIES – UNIQUE ROLES

Military families deal with a number of unique issues. However, a number of these issues have similarities to other families affected by psychological trauma.

Combat Deployment and the Family

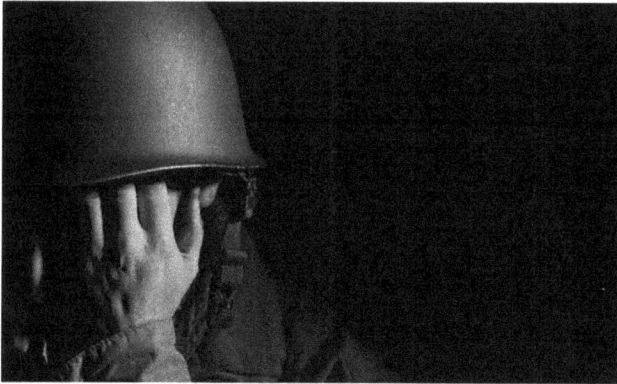

FIGURE 17: COMBAT DEPLOYMENT CAN TAKE A HEAVY TOLL ON THE SOLDIER

One thing military families usually have in common is that a parent and spouse has deployed to a foreign combat zone, most recently Iraq or Afghanistan. In today's military, families often have two, three, or four or more deployments, which is a significant change from the past.

I say the families deploy, because when the soldier deploys, it affects the whole family.

Understanding the psychological effects of deployment and combat trauma on the family is important to helping the family cope as a whole. These observations are based on experiences with a ten-day intensive program we developed for military families at the Callaway Gardens in Pine Mountain, Georgia, which I talk more about below.

The Wars in Iraq and Afghanistan

At the peak of the war in Iraq and Afghanistan—Operation Iraqi Freedom/Operation Enduring Freedom (OIF/OEF)–over 150,000 soldiers were deployed each year to the combat zone, and 12%-17% of them developed PTSD. In the State of Georgia alone, up to 13,000 soldiers returned each year from Iraq and Afghanistan. There were an equal number of direct family members in Georgia with a deployed spouse or parent in this time period. Many returning soldiers have been afflicted with a wide range of physical and mental health complaints.

Effects of Combat Deployment on Physical and Mental Health

Less than 40% of returning soldiers from OIF with PTSD will seek treatment for their disorder.

These military personnel will suffer from loss of work productivity, use more health care resources and have higher rates of disease, including cardiovascular disease (CVD), diabetes, asthma, PTSD and depression. Military personnel deployed in violent combat arenas have increased rates of impulsive and risk taking behavior, as well as increased violence and aggression upon returning from deployment, compared to non-deployed military personnel. They also have more physical symptoms, mental health problems, and alcohol and substance abuse.

Most alarming are the statistics related to the rise of suicide. The number of suicides in active duty military personnel and reserves increased from 160 in 2001 to 309 in 2009. The number of completed suicides was even higher in 2010, according to the Department of Defense.

In my opinion an important factor that contributes to suicide is a sense of anger and alienation upon return from combat deployments. Returning soldiers have trouble re-integrating into their communities and families. That's why in working with military families we always focus on family first.

The Cost of Deployment-related Mental Health Problems

Not addressing the consequences of stress related to deployment to combat zones is associated with significant costs. Among veterans of the Vietnam War, 23% percent of those with PTSD were not working in the years after returning from deployment, compared to 4% percent without PTSD.

The cost of lost productivity based on a rate of PTSD of 15% in the three million veterans who served in Vietnam and had an average salary of $30,000 over forty years is thus over $3.6 trillion dollars.

A RAND report from 2008 ("Stop loss: A nation weighs the tangible consequences of invisible combat wounds.") estimated the two-year year cost of PTSD and depression in terms of treatment, lost productivity and loss of life due to suicide in 1.6 million soldiers returning from Iraq and Afghanistan at $4-6.2 billion depending on how suicides are accounted for.

Individual costs per service member are

- $10,298 for PTSD,

- $16,884 for co-morbid PTSD and depression, and

- $25,757 for depression.

Furthermore, $1.7 billion ($2306 per case of PTSD, $2997 for PTSD/depression, and $9240 for depression) could be saved by treating all service members with these conditions. Extrapolated over forty years of additional lifetime, assuming that these conditions become chronic in half of persons, the dollar amount would be over $40 billion.

Effects of Combat Deployment on Military Families

The families of returning soldiers are also affected by their war time experiences.

Studies have shown that the families of veterans with combat-related PTSD exhibit more adjustment problems than the families of combat veterans who do not develop PTSD.

Families with a PTSD affected veteran were more likely to be rated as high on a Marital Problems Index (49% versus 9%),

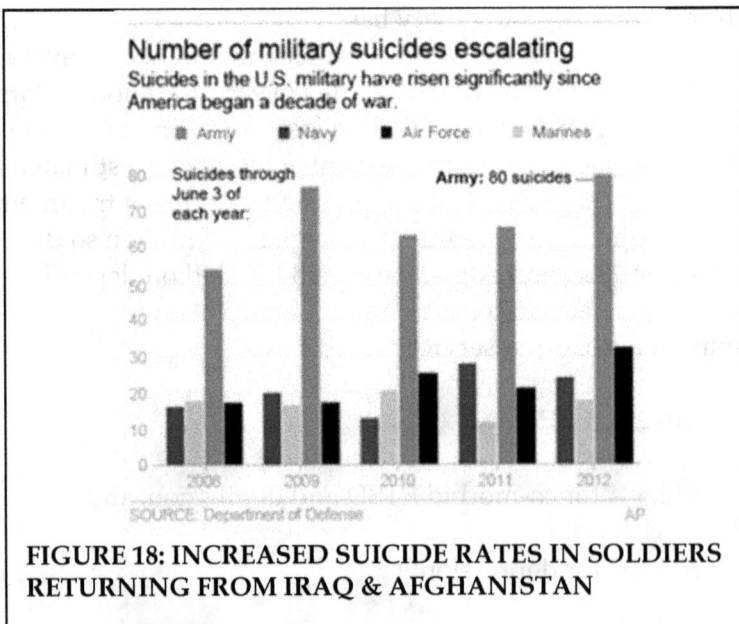

FIGURE 18: INCREASED SUICIDE RATES IN SOLDIERS RETURNING FROM IRAQ & AFGHANISTAN

- Parental Problem Index (55% versus 17%), and

- family adjustment (extreme) (55% versus 19%).

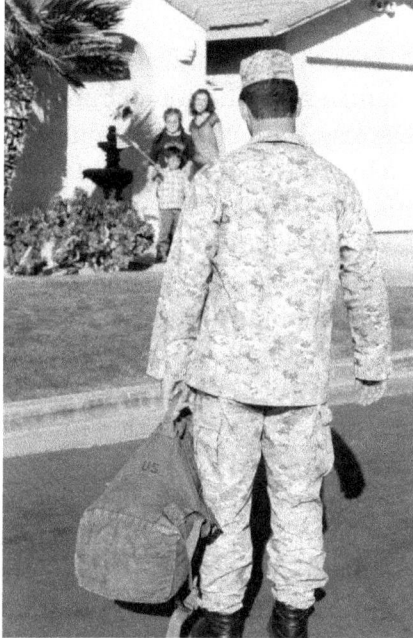

**FIGURE 19: THE SOLDIER
RETURNS HOME**

The rates of mental disorders in spouses who remain stateside are similar to those of their spouses deployed in a combat zone. Divorce rates have increased from 2.6% in 2001 to 3.6% in 2009 in military families, according to the Department of Defense. Children with deployed parents compared to those with non-deployed military parents suffer mental disorders at the rate of 20% versus 16% for boys, and 16% versus 14% for girls.

A Program for Re-integration of Soldiers into Family and Community

Soldiers are prepared by the military for deployment, but not necessarily for their return from the combat zone. Combat zones are associated with high stress, high physical demands, high adrenaline, high leadership and a high level of job sophistication.

Return from deployment feels like a rapid deceleration for soldiers, with an associated relative lack of activity, and if they are discharged from active duty service, possibly no job. Some soldiers are not ready for the return home and post-deployment period. Multiple forces converge that threaten connection with the soldier's family, work, and environment.

We decided that a program was needed for soldiers when they return from deployment, where they could spend time with their families in a relaxed outdoor environment, and learn about stress and gain additional skills related to diet, health, and relationships, as well as reconnect with their families, peers, and the natural environment.

In April and July of 2012, our research program at the Emory University School of Medicine, in conjunction with the US Army Maneuver Center of Excellence at Fort Benning in Columbus, Georgia, the Callaway family (Edward and Bo Callaway) and the Callaway Gardens Foundation conducted two ten-day pilot programs at the Callaway Gardens for soldiers returning from Iraq and Afghanistan and their families. The program was designed to facilitate re-integration of soldiers into their families, their communities, nature, and with each other. We called our program the Callaway Homecoming Initiative (CHI).

The mission of CHI was to help returning soldiers and their families learn about the symptoms of stress and the transition from the combat theater, become educated about health, diet, exercise, relationships, and personal life skills, adjust to life at home, and re-connect with nature, peers and family.

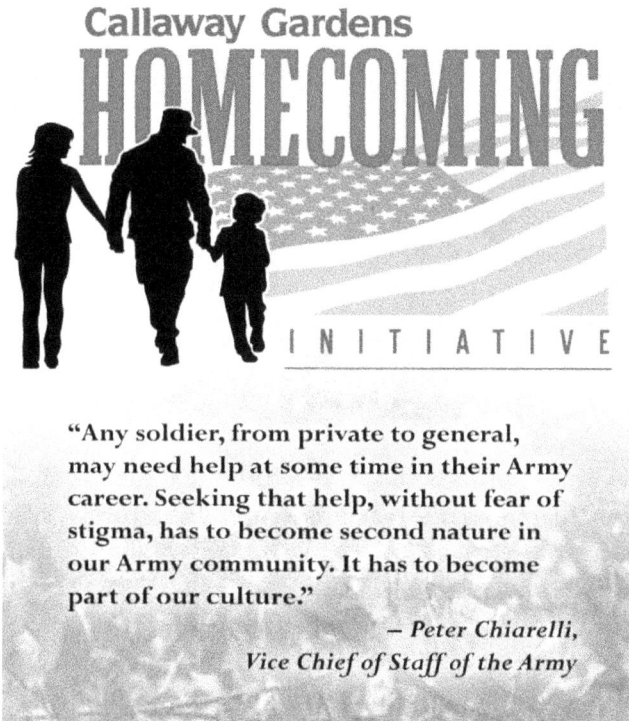

Callaway Gardens

HOMECOMING

INITIATIVE

"Any soldier, from private to general, may need help at some time in their Army career. Seeking that help, without fear of stigma, has to become second nature in our Army community. It has to become part of our culture."

— *Peter Chiarelli,*
Vice Chief of Staff of the Army

FIGURE 20: CALLAWAY HOMECOMING INITIATIVE (CHI) PROGRAM BROCHURE

Program for soldiers returning from Iraq and Afghanistan and their families, 2012. Copyright © 2012 Callaway Gardens, used by permission of Callaway Gardens.

This was done through a ten-day residential period for soldiers who had just returned from deployment and their immediate families in the environment of the Callaway Gardens, a 10,000-acre complex with cabins for the families, gardens, a nature center, golf, tennis and sailing, and a variety of family-oriented activities like zip lines and organized team competitions.

We included married soldiers who recently returned from deployment to a combat zone. We found that facilitating the coming together of families in an environment where individual family members can share their experiences with each other and their peers who can relate to their similar experiences was very helpful in promoting the re-integration of service members into their families and communities.

Our experience with this program was highly positive, with one spouse telling us that her soldier husband and she had decided to divorce, but changed their minds after going through the program.

This program helped not only the soldier, but also the spouse and children who were spared the devastating break-up of the family.

Stages of Deployment

Soldiers and their families go through multiple psychological stages before, during, and after deployment to a combat zone. These stages include:

- pre-deployment (the month or so before leaving),

- initial deployment (the first month in the combat zone),

- sustainment (the middle portion of deployment),

- re-deployment (two months before return), and

- the post-deployment period.

The <u>pre-deployment</u> period represents the time leading up to deployment.

The soldier may seem "already deployed" since he is focused on his unit and getting ready. There is an endless "to do" list before the soldier deploys.

It is not uncommon to have a "big argument" with the spouse—more likely related to stress than fundamental problems in the marriage. But the soldier may deploy before there is time to make up and come to a mutual understanding.

In general, there may not be a chance to tie up loose ends. Kids are getting ready for the adjustment of not having two parents in the house, and worried about what will happen to their soldier/parent.

Some spouses admit that there is so much tension leading up to "the time" when the soldier actually leaves that they almost feel a sense of relief when it's over. Many spouses we met with in our groups admitted this and felt relieved that others felt the same way, since they had not talked about it before because they felt guilty.

The underline deployment period refers to the first month of deployment overseas.

Spouses at home may have trouble adjusting to not having the spouse in bed, or someone around the house to help out. They have to get used to being single parents. The kids need to adjust to not having an extra parent.

Many military spouses seem to learn to do a number of things that non-military spouses don't do; for example, it might be typical that one spouse controls the finances and pays the bills, while the other one doesn't know anything about it. Military families don't have this luxury, so they evolve as two parallel units that are both self-sufficient. This may be associated with its own problems.

Sustainment refers to the period when everyone settles into the routine of the soldier being away from home for a long period of time, i.e., the months in the middle of the deployment, after the soldier and family have gotten used to him or her not being there, and before they start psychologically getting ready for their return a couple of months before the end of the deployment period.

During this period, the spouse on the home front goes through a period of endlessly waiting for the phone to ring — a never-ending dread by the spouse and the kids that they will get the phone call, or the visit to the door, telling them that their parent and spouse has been killed in combat.

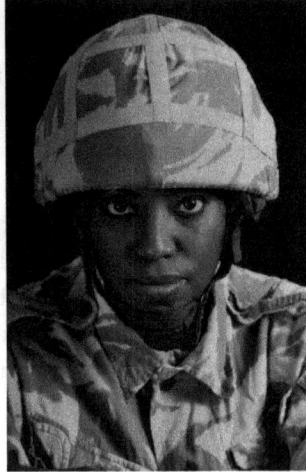

**FIGURE 21: AN
INCREASING NUMBER
OF OUR MILITARY
ARE WOMEN**

Some spouses report sleeping with their cell phones on their chest, because they never know when the call will come in, day or night, and they may not get the chance to call back.

Sometimes when the call does come, it can be frustrating, because they have to drop everything they are doing to attend to the soldier. They may feel like there is no appreciation for the fact that they have their own life that is not less important than what is happening in the combat zone.

Sometimes well-intentioned efforts to support military families can backfire and themselves become the source of stress. The Family Readiness Groups (FRGs) are networks of spouses with soldiers in the same unit that were formed with the goal of providing mutual support. However, rumors can quickly spread.

When there is a casualty or the unit goes out on a combat mission, there is a blackout of information for security reasons. During the period (which may be up to two days) the spouses cannot communicate with their partners. In this environment rumors can spread. We have met at least one spouse who thought that her partner was killed in action based on rumors in the FRG, when in fact her spouse was unharmed.

Rumors can also spread about infidelity and other issues. For these reasons, rumors should be brought out into the open as soon as possible so that they can be quelled.

The re-deployment period refers to the month or two before the soldier returns home.

This is an adjustment period both for the soldier and for the family members on the home front. The spouse may panic over the list of things to do to prepare for the return of the soldiers.

Sometimes the spouse may not "be ready" for the return of the soldier.

Post-deployment starts with the initial joy and anxiety of re-unitement—most couples and their children report great joy at the initial reunion.

Once the soldier is back in the house, however, it may take time to adjust. Sometimes the soldier wants to indulge his kids, or introduces changes in the rules for the kids which frustrates the other spouse who has been holding to boundaries about things like bedtime or video time.

The spouse may have to get used to having someone else in the house. The new parent may have his or her own ideas of discipline for the kids. It may take some time to adjust.

Small children may experience some fear at seeing a parent they don't remember. Often small children see their deployed parent as someone who lives in the computer, since their contact with them up to that point has been through Skype or the telephone. Some of the families in our program printed out life-size full-length photographs of the deployed parent and made "cardboard cut-out daddies" to help the kids have something to represent the missing parent.

When that parent returns and wants them to sit on their laps, it can be a little scary at first and may require some period for adjustment.

Coming Home

When a soldier comes back from the combat front, s/he can't just

NEURAL ACTIVITY IN THE FIGHT-OR-FLIGHT RESPONSE

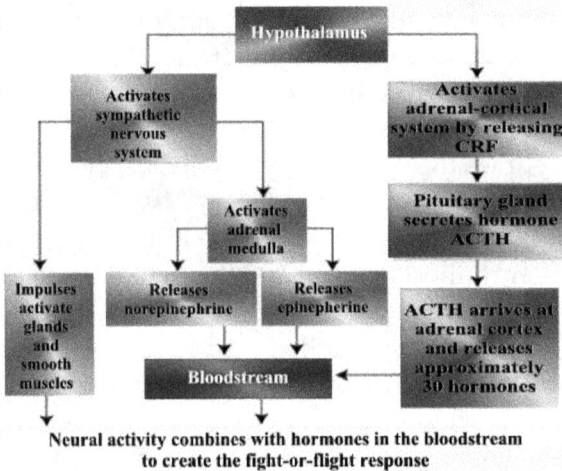

Neural activity combines with hormones in the bloodstream
to create the fight-or-flight response

**FIGURE 22: NEUROPHYSIOLOGIC ACTIVITY
IN THE FIGHT OR FLIGHT RESPONSE**

"turn off" their combat frame of mind the way you flick a switch to turn off the light. Soldiers in a combat zone have a heightened responsiveness and increased vigilance.

Being hyped up and on guard is a normal and adaptive response to being in a combat zone. Soldiers who didn't stay on their toes might be at risk to get picked off by a sniper or to not respond fast enough to an ambush. In that case, they'd be coming back in a body bag instead of an airplane.

The "fight or flight response" facilitates survival in combat. As discussed earlier in this book, stress hormones adrenaline and cortisol pour into the body when there is a threat and cause an increase in heart rate, blood pressure, and breathing rate, and shunt energy to the muscles and brain so you think fast, run fast, and fight hard.

Since the combat mode is an automatic response (if you had to think too much about it, you probably wouldn't survive) it isn't something that can just be "willed" away.

That's why soldier's families shouldn't be impatient if their soldiers are jumpy or on guard when they get back from the war zone, and that their jumpiness doesn't go away right away.

THE PHYSIOLOGY OF FIGHT OR FLIGHT

What we know is happening...

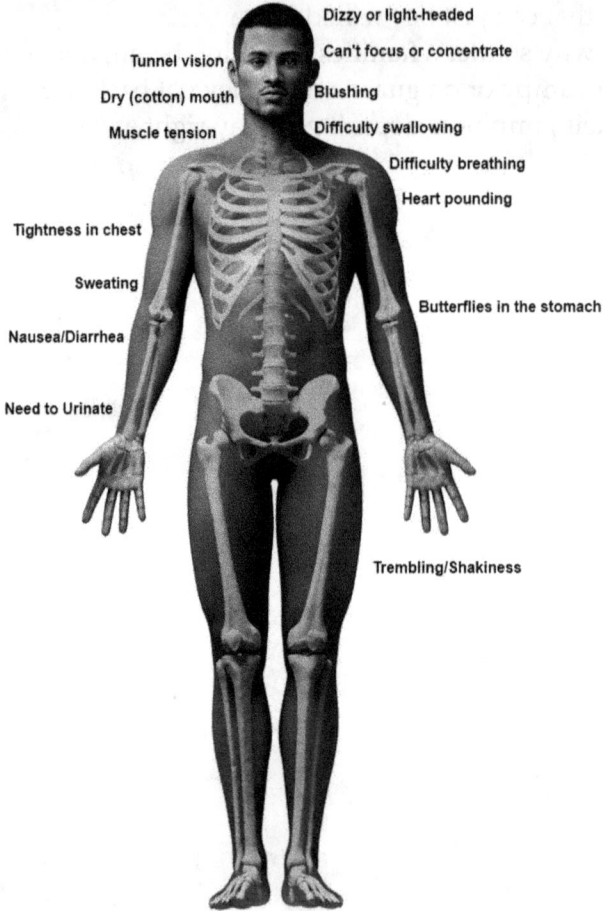

FIGURE 23: THE PHYSIOLOGY OF FLIGHT OR FIGHT

Learned Combat-Zone Behaviors Don't Translate Well to Civilian Life

Soldiers learn other behaviors to adapt in a combat zone that may seem strange after they come home.

In Iraq, soldiers drove their armored vehicles at full bore down the middle of the road. If there were some vehicles in front of them, they would pass like maniacs, even if it meant putting everyone at risk. They did that because explosive devices were left at the side of the road in garbage bags or other hidden places.

These "improvised explosive devices" (or IEDs) were detonated remotely by insurgents when the soldiers were on patrol. If they got slowed down by other vehicles or by crowds of civilians in the road, they became easy targets for IEDs. That's why they learned how to drive fast and furious when they were on patrol.

Back home, a simple drive to the grocery store can become a frightening experience. They also can drive other people crazy — they'll often honk at little old ladies who they think are driving too slow or getting in the way. Seeing a bag of garbage on the side of the road can cause them to swerve.

When the Combat Mind Interferes with Living

The difficulty in turning off the combat mind set may come out in other ways:

- Soldiers may stay at home to avoid things that trigger memories of combat. They may feel safer.

- They may get anxious when their loved ones go out as well.

- They may jump at loud noises.

- Sleeping with someone else in bed may feel strange.

- Being a parent, and making decisions will be a challenge.

- For many soldiers, it is the first time out of the military, and they must learn how to get a job, balance a checkbook, shop for groceries, cook for themselves (instead of eating on base), clean the house, and be a parent.

- Wives and kids must adjust to having another person in the house.

The Callaway Homecoming Initiative (CHI)

The Callaway Homecoming Initiative (CHI) was focused on reintegrating soldiers with their families.

For the first few days of the program, soldiers came in by themselves. In the mornings, they got a series of lectures from mental health experts on mental and physical health, relationships, better lifestyles and transitioning from the combat theater. Afternoons were spent in team building activities.

After several days, we brought in the families, and had a lecture on unique role of military spouses just for the spouses, followed by a group discussion and a team building activity in the afternoon. The next day we gave lectures to the couples on working together as couples, and did similar things for the kids.

The program let soldiers spend time with their spouses and children in a setting that allowed them to learn and grow together, have positive shared experiences, and participate in activities that allowed them to reconnect with nature and bond together as families.

The lessons we learned from the program apply to all families where one or more people are affected by psychological trauma. We learned that one of the most important factors in the recovery from psychological trauma is the love and support of the family members.

When soldiers, or anyone for that matter, become detached from their families, it leads to anger, isolation, despair, and ultimately suicide.

In recognition of the important role of family members, we have written the next chapter for the significant others and spouses of those affected by psychological trauma.

CHAPTER 14: MOVING BEYOND TRAUMA

As you work with your client who suffers from psychological trauma it is important to keep your eye on the bigger picture. They may suffer setbacks and feel worse at times, but they stick with it they will ultimately get there. Remind them that they are actively doing something about their trauma, as opposed to other family members who dealt with it by avoidance, and that they are moving toward a place that will ultimately be better for their families.

For all patients, recovery is a long and often circular process. Ultimately when your clients start to recover from their trauma, suggest to them the possibility of making something positive out of their experience. Perhaps being a Big Brother, or volunteering in the community. I often tell my clients who are of a religious faith to talk to their pastor or minister about places they can volunteer. They can use their experiences in recovery from trauma to help others who are less fortunate. Doing something for others counteracts negative cognitions that the world is a terrible place. It also gives them an outlet to connect with other people, get out of the house, become less isolated and socialize with other people. All of these things are ultimately positive for patients who have experienced psychological trauma.

ABOUT THE AUTHOR

J. Douglas Bremner, M.D.

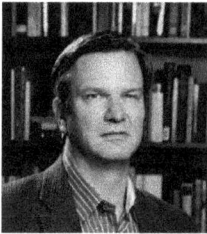

J. Douglas Bremner, M.D. is Professor of Psychiatry and Radiology and Director of the Emory Clinical Neuroscience Research Unit (ECNRU) at Emory University School of Medicine and the Atlanta VA Medical Center in Atlanta, Georgia. He spends one day a week seeing soldiers returning from Iraq and Afghanistan and performing assessments on other veterans with mental health complaints.

He has a long history of experience in the field of PTSD and trauma dating back to his role as the Medical Director of the first inpatient unit for PTSD at the National Center for PTSD in West Haven, Connecticut. His research on changes in the brain and symptoms of trauma, dissociation, and PTSD are amongst the most highly cited in his field.

He is the author of several best-selling books including *Does Stress Damage the Brain?* and *Before You Take That Pill* as well as the personal narrative *The Goose that Laid the Golden Egg*.

Dr. Bremner lives in Atlanta, Georgia.

APPENDIX A: EMOTIONAL WORDS

Afraid	Alive	Angry	Apprehensive
Ashamed	Awkward	Bitter	Brave
Calm	Capable	Competent	Concerned
Confused	Contemptuous	Courageous	Defeated
Dejected	Dependent	Depressed	Despairing
Desperate	Devastated	Disappointed	Discouraged
Disgusted	Distrustful	Embarrassed	Exasperated
Fearful	Foolish	Forgiving	Frantic
Frustrated	Furious	Guilty	Hateful
Helpless	Hopeless	Horrified	Hostile
Humiliated	Hurt	Ignored	Impatient
Inadequate	Incompetent	Indecisive	Inferior
Inhibited	Insecure	Irritated	Isolated
Jealous	Lonely	Melancholy	Miserable
Misunderstood	Muddled	Needy	Neglected
Old	Outraged	Overwhelmed	Panicky
Peaceful	Pessimistic	Phony	Preoccupied
Pressured	Provoked	Quiet	Relaxed
Relieved	Regretful	Rejected	Resentful
Revengeful	Sad	Self-conscious	Self-reliant
Shy	Sorry	Strong	Stubborn
Stupid	Terrified	Threatened	Tired
Touchy	Trapped	Troubled	Unappreciated
Unattractive	Uncertain	Uncomfortable	Uneasy
Unfulfilled	Used	Uptight	Victimized
Violated	Vulnerable	Weary	Wishy-washy
Worn-out	Worried		

APPENDIX B: RESOURCES FOR TRAUMA VICTIMS

National Center for Victims of Crime. 1-800-FYI-CALL. This is a comprehensive database of more than 6,700 community service agencies throughout the country that directly support victims of crime.

Trauma Treatment. For veterans, look under Health Benefits and Services at www.va.gov. If not, look in the "County Government Offices" section of the phone book under your county and look for "Health Services" and "Mental Health."

Anxiety Disorders of America (ADAA). The ADAA has a referral network of therapists including a list of PTSD experts, as well as a self-help network. I personally approve their recommendations for self-help books, so your clients can go to their on-line book store for their self-help book selections. I think it is a good idea to buy self-help books and try to follow them. www.adaa.org.

The *National Institute of Mental Health (NIMH)* is a great resource for information. Your clients can learn a lot about trauma by looking at www.nih.gov.

The *National Center for PTSD* is where I spent the first part of my career treating patients and doing research in PTSD. Their web site has some great information. Research articles are also included, if you want to read them, you can download them. ncptsd.org

Sidran Press is a great place for books about trauma. They also have a list of professional referrals. www.sidran.org

David Baldwin has a great web page that has a wealth of information about trauma, resources, information and treatment. He is a clinical psychologist in Eugene, Oregon. www.trauma-pages.com

The Oldways Preservation and Exchange Trust is a nonprofit foundation dedicated to promotion of the Mediterranean Diet and other healthy behaviors. http://oldwayspt.org

National Domestic Abuse Hotline: 1–800–799–SAFE (7233) or TTY 1-800-787-3224.

National Child Abuse Hotline: 1-800-4-A-CHILD (1-800-422-4453)

Eldercare Help Locator (not 24 hours) 1-800-677-1116

APPENDIX C: LIST OF IMAGES AND DIAGRAMS

(permissions, sources and credits)

Figure 1.   Hippocampal volume in PTSD

From figure 4.2 in *Does Stress Damage the Brain? Understanding Trauma-related Disorders from a Mind-Body Perspective*, by J. Douglas Bremner. Copyright © 2002 by J. Douglas Bremner, M.D. Used by permission of W. W. Norton & Company, Inc.

Figure 2.   Trauma Spectrum Disorder

Adapted from *Does Stress Damage the Brain? Understanding Trauma-related Disorders from a Mind-Body Perspective*, by J. Douglas Bremner. Copyright © 2002 by J. Douglas Bremner, M.D. Used by permission of W. W. Norton & Company, Inc.

Figure 3.   DSM-IV-TR Criteria for Major Depression

© 2014 J. Douglas Bremner, adapted from DSM-IV-TR APA. (2000). *DSM-IV-TR: Diagnostic and Statistical Manual of Mental Disorders*. Washington, D.C.: American Psychiatric Press.

Figure 4.   DSM-IV-TR Criteria for Post Traumatic Stress Disorder (PTSD)

Adapted from DSM-IV-TR APA. (2000). *DSM-IV-TR: Diagnostic and Statistical Manual of Mental Disorders*. Washington, D.C.: American Psychiatric Press.

Figure 5.   Diagram of the Human Brain

Retrieved from Wikipedia, free use.

Figure 6.   Surface of the Human Brain

Retrieved from Wikipedia, free use.

Figure 7.   Neurohormonal Responses to Stress

From figure 3.3 in *Does Stress Damage the Brain? Understanding Trauma-related Disorders from a Mind-Body Perspective*, by J. Douglas Bremner. Copyright © 2002 by J. Douglas Bremner, M.D. Used by permission of W. W. Norton & Company, Inc.

Figure 8.   The Neuron: Basic Cell of the Human Brain

Used with permission of Hollowtree Workshops © 2014

Figure 9.   Brain activation with exposure to traumatic reminders

From figure 4.5 in *Does Stress Damage the Brain? Understanding Trauma-related Disorders from a Mind-Body Perspective*, by J. Douglas Bremner. Copyright © 2002 by J. Douglas Bremner, M.D. Used by permission of W. W. Norton & Company, Inc.

Figure 10.   Need to Escape

By Igor Petrov via license from Shutterstock.

Figure 11.   Stages of Grief

By Marekulasz via license from Shutterstock

Figure 12.   Antidepressant Medications – Uses and Risks

From BEFORE YOU TAKE THAT PILL, by J. Douglas Bremner, © 2008 J. Douglas Bremner, used by permission of Avery Publishing, an imprint of the Penguin Group.

Figure 13.   Antipsychotic Medications: Uses and Risks
From BEFORE YOU TAKE THAT PILL, by J. Douglas Bremner, © 2008 J. Douglas Bremner, used by permission of Avery Publishing, an imprint of the Penguin Group. Public domain.

Figure 14.   Insomnia Medications: Uses and Risks

From BEFORE YOU TAKE THAT PILL, by J. Douglas Bremner, © 2008 J. Douglas Bremner, used by permission of Avery Publishing, an imprint of the Penguin Group.

Figure 15.   Mediterranean Diet food pyramid

Used with permission of Oldways Preservation and Exchange Trust. http://oldwayspt.org. Copyright © 2012 Oldways Preserva-tion and Exchange Trust.

Figure 16.   Symptoms of Alcohol & Substance Abuse

© 2014 J. Douglas Bremner, adapted from DSM-IV-TR APA. (2000). *DSM-IV-TR: Diagnostic and Statistical Manual of Mental Disorders.* Washington, D.C.: American Psychiatric Press.

Figure 17.   Combat Deployment Can Take a Heavey Toll on the Soldier

By John Gomez via Shutterstock

Figure 18.   Increased Suicide Rates in Soldiers Returning from Iraq and Afghanistan

Figure from thinkprogress.org, source of information Department of Defence. Copyright   © 2012 Center for American Progress Action Fund (CAPAF). Accessed 8/10/13 from http://thinkprogress.org/security/2012/06/08/496604/military-suicide/

Figure 19.   The Soldier Returns Home

By bikeriderlondon via Shutterstock

Figure 20.   Callaway Homecoming Initiative brochure

Copyright © 2012 Callaway Gardens, used by permission of Callaway Gardens.

Figure 21.   An Increasing Number of Our Military are Women

By John Gomez via Shutterstock

Figure 22.   Neurophysiologic Activity in the Fight or Flight Response

Used with permission of Hollowtree Workshops © 2014

Figure 23.   The Physiology of Fight-or-Flight Reactions

By Sebastian Kaulitzki via Shutterstock.

APPENDIX D: BIBLIOGRAPHY AND RECOMMENDED READING

American Psychiatric Association. *DSM-IV-TR: Diagnostic and Statistical Manual of Mental Disorders.* American Psychiatric Press, Washington, D.C. 2000.

Bremner, J.D., Southwick, S.M., Brett, E., Fontana, A., Rosenheck, A., Charney, D.S. Dissociation and posttraumatic stress disorder in Vietnam combat veterans. *American Journal of Psychiatry.* 1992; 149:328-332.

Bremner, J.D., Southwick, S.M., Johnson, D.R., Yehuda, R., Charney, D.S. Childhood physical abuse and combat-related posttraumatic stress disorder in Vietnam veterans. *American Journal of Psychiatry.* 1993; 150:235-239.

Bremner, J. D., Southwick, S.M., Darnell, A., Charney, D.S. Chronic PTSD in Vietnam combat veterans: Course of illness and substance abuse. *American Journal of Psychiatry.* 1996; 153:369-375.

Bremner, J.D., Vermetten, E., & Mazure, C.M. Development and preliminary psychometric properties of an instrument for the measurement of childhood trauma: The Early Trauma Inventory. *Depression and Anxiety.* 2000; 12:1-12.

Bremner, J. Douglas. *Does Stress Damage the Brain? Understanding Trauma-related Disorders from a Mind-Body Perspective.* WW Norton, New York, NY, 2002.

Bremner, J. Douglas. *Brain Imaging Handbook.* WW Norton, New York, NY, 2005.

Bremner, J. Douglas. *Before You Take that Pill: Why the Drug Industry May Be Bad For Your Health: Risks and Side Effects You Won't Find on the Label of Commonly Prescribed Drugs and Supplements.* Avery/Penguin, New York, NY, 2008.

Bremner, J. Douglas. Combat-related Psychiatric Syndromes. In: *Functional Pain Syndromes: Presentation and Pathophysiology.* Mayer,

Emeran A., and Bushnell M.C. (Eds.); Seattle, WA, US: IASP Press, 2009. pp. 169-183.

Bremner, Doug. *The Goose That Laid the Golden Egg — Accutane, the truth that had to be told.* Right Publishing, San Francisco, CA, 2011.

Bremner, Doug. *The Fastest Growing Religion on Earth: How Genealogy Captured the Brains and Imaginations of Americans.* Laughing Cow Books, Atlanta, GA, 2013.

Bremner, J. Douglas. Emory Clinical Neuroscience Research Unit (ECNRU) web site, http://www.psychiatry.emory.edu/research/laboratories/bremner/index.html accessed September 14, 2014.

Briere, John. *Child Abuse Trauma: Theory and Treatment of the Lasting Effects.* Sage Publications, Newbury Park, CA, 1992.

Brondolo, Elizabeth, and Xavier Amador. *Break the Bipolar Cycle: A Day-by-Day Guide to Living with Bipolar Disorder.* McGraw-Hill Books, New York, 2008.

Brown, Nina W. *Children of the Self-Absorbed: A Grown Up's Guide to Getting Over Narcissistic Parents.* 2nd Edition. New Harbinger Publications, Oakland, CA, 2008.

Cyrulnik, Boris. *The Whispering of Ghosts: Trauma and Resilience.* Other Press, New York, 2005.

Donaldson-Pressman, Stephanie, and Robert M. Pressman. *The Narcissistic Family: Diagnosis and Treatment.* Josey-Bass, New York, 1997.

Erichsen, John Eric. *On Railway and Other Injuries of the Nervous System.* Henry C. Lee, Philadelphia PA, 1867.

Freud, Anna. *Ego and the Mechanisms of Defense.* International Universities Press, New York, 1965.

Freud, Sigmund. *Introductory Lectures on Psychoanalysis.* WW Norton, New York, 1965.

Freud, Sigmund. *The Interpretation of Dreams.* Avon, New York, 1965.

Freyd, Jennifer J. *Betrayal Trauma: The logic of forgetting childhood abuse.* Harvard Press, Cambridge, Mass., 1996.

Gabriel, Richard A. *No More Heroes: Madness and Psychiatry in War.* Hill and Wang, New York, 1987.

Herman, Judith. *Trauma and Recovery: The aftermath of violence – from domestic abuse to political terror.* Basic Books, New York, 1997.

Jung, Carl G. *Man and His Symbols.* Dell Nonfiction, New York, 1964.

Kabat-Zinn, Jon. *Full Catastrophic Living: Using the Wisdom of your Body and Mind to Face Stress, Pain, and Illness.* Delta Health Psychology, New York, 1990.

Kessler, R.C., Sonnega, A., Bromet, E., Hughes, M., Nelson, C.B. Posttraumatic stress disorder in the national comorbidity survey. *Archives of General Psychiatry.* 1995;52:1048-1060.

Kessler, R.C., Berglund, P., Demler, O., Jin, R., Koretz, D., Merikangas, K.R., Rush, A.J., Walters, E.E., Wang, P.S. The epidemiology of major depressive disorder: Results from the national comorbidity survey replication (ncs-r). *JAMA.* 2003;289:3095-3105

Kirmayer, L. J., Lemelson, R., & Barad, M. (Eds.). *Understanding Trauma: Integrating Biological, Clinical and Cultural Perspectives.* Cambridge University Press, Cambridge, United Kingdom, 2007.

Kubler-Ross, Elisabeth. *On Death and Dying.* Scribner, New York, 1969.

Langs, Robert. *Rating Your Psychotherapist: Find out whether your therapy is working – and what to do if it's not.* Henry Holt, New York, 1989.

LeDoux, Joseph. *The Emotional Brain: The mysterious underpinnings of emotional life.* Simon & Schuster, New York, 1996.

Levine, Peter A. *Waking the Tiger: Healing Trauma.* North Atlantic Books, Berkeley, CA, 1997.

Mehl-Madrona, Lewis. *Healing the Mind through the Power of Story: The Promise of Narrative Psychiatry.* Bear & Company, Rochester, VT, 2010.

Middelton-Moz, Jane. *Shame and Guilt: Masters of Disguise.* Health Communications, Inc., Deerfield Beach, FL, 1990.

Miller, Alice. *The Drama of the Gifted Child: How Narcissistic Parents Form and Deform the Emotional Lives of Their Talented Children.* Basic Book, New York, 1981.

Miller, Alice. *Prisoners of Chilhood: The Drama of the Gifted Child and the Search for the True Self.* Basic Book, New York, 1987.

Ross, Colin. *Dissociative Identity Disorder: Diagnosis, Clinical Features, and Treatment of Multiple Personality*. Wiley Press, New York, 1996

Ross, Colin. *The Great Psychiatry Scam: One Shrink's Personal Journey*. Manitou Press, Richardson, Texas, 2008.

Ross, Colin and Naomi Halpern. *Trauma Model Therapy: A treatment approach for trauma, dissociation and complex comorbidity*. Manitou Communications, Richardson, Texas, 1989.

Ross, Colin. *The Trauma Model: A Solution to the Problem of Comorbidity in Psychiatry*. Manitou Press, Richardson, Texas, 2000.

Saigh, Phillip; Bremner, J. Douglas (Editors): *Posttraumatic Stress Disorder: A Comprehensive Text.* Allyn & Bacon, Needham Heights, MA, 1999.

Schlesinger, Laura: *Cope with it!* Kensington Press, New York, 2000.

Shay, Jonathan. *Achilles and Vietnam: Combat Trauma and the Undoing of Character*. Simon & Schuster, New York, 1995.

Siegel, Daniel J. *The Developing Mind: Toward a Neurobiology of Interpersonal Experience*. Guilford Press, New York, 1999.

Stewart, W.F., Ricci, J.A., Chee, E., Hahn, S.R., Morganstein, D. Cost of lost productive work time among us workers with depression. *JAMA*. 2003;289:3135-3144.

Terr, Lenore: *Too Scared to Cry: How Trauma Affects Children... and Ultimately Us All*. Basic Books, New York, 1990.

Vaccarino, Viola, and Bremner, J. Douglas. Cardiovascular disease and depression. In: *Braunwald's Heart Disease*, 2011.

van der Kolk, Bessel. *Psychological Trauma*. APA Press, Washington DC, 1987.

van der Kolk, Bessel. *The Body Keeps the Score: Brain, Mind and Body in the Healing of Psychological Trauma*. Viking Adult, 2014.

Wachs, Kim M. *Relationships for Dummies*. Wiley, 2002.

Whitfield, Charles L. *A Gift to Myself: A Personal Workbook and Guide to the Bestselling 'Healing the Child Within'*. Health Communications Inc., Deerfield Beach, FL, 1987.

Whitfield, Charles L. *Healing the Child Within*. Health Communications Inc., Deerfield Beach, FL, 1987.

Whitfield, Charles L. *The Truth About Mental Illness.* Health Communications Inc., Deerfield Beach, FL, 2004.

Whitmore-Hickman, Martha. *Healing After Loss: Daily Meditations for Recovery from Grief.*

Winnicott, Donald. *The Family and Individual Development.* Tavistock Press, Tavistock, Mass., 1965.

Wolfe, Thomas. *You Can't Go Home Again.* Scribner, New York, 2011.

INDEX

www.ingramcontent.com/pod-product-compliance
Lightning Source LLC
Chambersburg PA
CBHW071222290326
41931CB00037B/1853